Refractive Surgery - Types of Procedures, Risks, and Benefits

Edited by Maja Bohač and Mateja Jagić

Published in London, United Kingdom

Refractive Surgery - Types of Procedures, Risks, and Benefits
http://dx.doi.org/10.5772/intechopen.98100
Edited by Maja Bohač and Mateja Jagić

Contributors
Fanka Gilevska, Maja Bohač, Mateja Jagić, Smiljka Popović Suić, Pavol Vesely, Kamila Kopálová, Daniel Laroche, Kara Rickford, Iva Dekaris, Ivan Gabric, Doria Gabrić, Lucija Zerjav

First published in London, United Kingdom, 2022 by IntechOpen
IntechOpen is the global imprint of INTECHOPEN LIMITED, registered in England and Wales, registration number: 11086078, 5 Princes Gate Court, London, SW7 2QJ, United Kingdom

British Library Cataloguing-in-Publication Data
A catalogue record for this book is available from the British Library

Additional hard and PDF copies can be obtained from orders@intechopen.com

Refractive Surgery - Types of Procedures, Risks, and Benefits
Edited by Maja Bohač and Mateja Jagić
p. cm.
Print ISBN 978-1-80355-900-1
Online ISBN 978-1-80355-901-8
eBook (PDF) ISBN 978-1-80355-902-5

Meet the editors

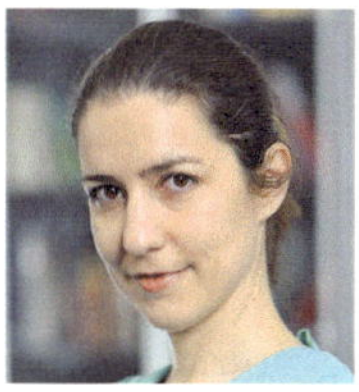

Maja Bohač graduated from the Faculty of Medicine at the University of Zagreb and specialized in ophthalmology under the mentorship of Professor Nikica Gabrić. Her postgraduate study of biomedicine and health was undertaken at the Faculty of Medicine of the University of Zagreb. In 2017 she obtained her doctorate with a dissertation on "Comparison of mechanical microkeratome and femtosecond lasers". She completed additional training in refractive surgery in London, Zurich, Barcelona, Cologne and Strasbourg and was appointed assistant professor at the Faculty of Medicine, University of Rijeka. As the head of the refractive surgery department at the University Eye Hospital Svjetlost, she is responsible for leading a team of ten refractive surgeons and for introducing new technologies in the field of laser refractive surgery. She has performed more than 30,000 laser surgeries, and specializes in complex cases such as scars, corneal damage and earlier refractive surgery. She is one of the first doctors in the region to use femtosecond lasers. She is also one of the first doctors to perform laser removal of presbyopia and has pioneered a new type of laser vision correction called SMILE and Smart Sight. She is a member of the International Society of Refractive Surgery, the European Society of Cataract and Refractive Surgery and the Croatian Society of Cataract and Refractive Surgery. She regularly participates as an active lecturer and educator at the annual meetings of these associations. Dr. Bohač has published 25 papers indexed in CC, of which the most important papers are related to the treatment of high astigmatism with excimer lasers.

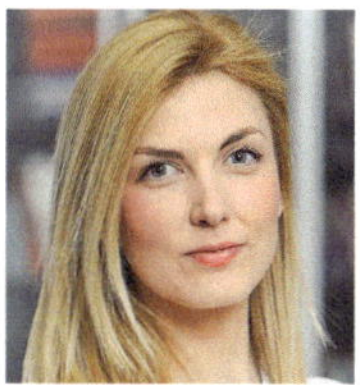

Mateja Jagić graduated from the Faculty of Medicine, at the University of Osijek, completing her specialization in ophthalmology and optometry in 2017 under the mentorship of Professor Iva Dekaris, and her postgraduate study in biomedicine and health at the Faculty of Medicine of the University of Zagreb. Her doctoral dissertation thesis was entitled "Visual outcome after implantation of multifocal intraocular lenses". Since 2011 she has worked in the Department of Refractive Surgery and the Corneal Department at the Specialty Hospital of Ophthalmology Svjetlost. Her training in corneal refractive surgery began under the mentorship of Assistant Professor Maja Bohač and so far, she has performed several thousand laser surgeries. Mateja Jagić is a member of the European Association for Cataract and Refractive Surgery and the Croatian Society for Cataract and Refractive Surgery and regularly participates in annual meetings. She is a co-author of several scientific and professional papers in international journals cited in CC and in the field of refractive surgery.

Contents

Preface

Refractive surgery, meaning any procedure that corrects or minimizes refractive errors, has gained popularity worldwide in recent decades. This book provides essential information about the refractive error most commonly encountered in clinical practice, myopia. Today, laser refractive surgery is recognized as an effective and safe procedure for correcting low and moderate refractive errors, and it has evolved beyond the traditional LASIK procedure. A systematic approach to potential complications is essential to enable refractive surgeons to improve visual outcomes and prevent vision-threatening problems. New keratorefractive techniques such as lenticular extraction (SMILE, SmartSight, CLEAR) are gaining popularity in clinical practice, showing excellent results compared to the standard LASIK technique, but avoiding flap creation and maintaining the biomechanical stability of the cornea.

The chapter on cataract surgery discusses recent progress in surgical techniques, the introduction of a variety of intraocular lenses, advanced optics and the management of specific cases, including options for refractive correction in patients with high residual refractive errors after keratoplasty. With the merging of technologies evolving in the two ophthalmic subspecialties of cataract and glaucoma surgery, good refractive results with minimal spectacle dependence can now be achieved for glaucoma patients.

The goal of this book's editors has been to provide clinically relevant overviews incorporating new developments as well as future perspectives in the fields of refractive, cataract, and combined surgery. We hope that researchers, ophthalmology specialists, and trainees with an interest in refractive surgery will find it interesting and useful. Finally, we acknowledge the support of our outstanding authors, and the time and care they have devoted to their chapters to enable the completion of this book.

Maja Bohač and Mateja Jagić
Refractive Surgery Department,
University Eye Hospital Svjetlost,
Zagreb, Croatia

Section 1

Introduction

Chapter 1

Introductory Chapter: Refractive Surgery

Maja Bohač and Mateja Jagić

1. Introduction

Refractive surgery today includes surgical procedures by which it is possible to reduce or eliminate a certain type of refractive error [1]. To date, with advances in technology, it has evolved far beyond the standard keratorefractive surgery. Thanks to the development of femtosecond technology and lasers, the precision of the LASIK procedure has been raised to a new level, and new keratorefractive methods, such as SMILE, have been developed [2]. To address refractive errors in patients who do not meet the criteria for standard laser surgery, phakic lens implantation stands as a safe surgical treatment with the possibility of correcting extreme refractive errors. We also witnessed the development of surgical methods for the correction of presbyopia with new laser ablation profiles, intracorneal implants, and the introduction of new generations of presbyopia-correcting intraocular lenses (IOLs). Extensive developments in methods of corneal biomechanics and topography analysis have led to easier identification of patients who are potentially risky candidates due to the possible development of keratectasia [3, 4]. Currently, most ophthalmic practice works on the principle of validating preoperative data by physicians, while in the future we are likely to face an era of artificial intelligence and the implementation of machine learning as a more precise way of finding appropriate parameters or functions to classify input data from large amounts of training data. This would greatly simplify the method of detecting borderline candidates for keratorefractive procedure, discriminating keratoconus from normal corneas, and finding the best-suitable IOL for providing complete spectacle independence without compromising functional vision and optical quality [3–5].

2. Refractive surgery

2.1 Preoperative evaluation for refractive surgery

For patients seeking spectacle independence, detailed preoperative assessment plays a key role in determining a safe and effective outcome. Examination for refractive surgery begins with taking a detailed medical history that includes systemic status, medication, allergies, ocular status, and history of contact lens use. The examination itself consists of a detailed biomicroscopic examination of the anterior and posterior segments of the eye, and the measurement of intraocular pressure. Refraction is the most important part of the preoperative examination. Each patient needs to determine the manifest refraction, monocular uncorrected, and

IntechOpen

best-corrected visual acuity at distance and near. In addition to the examination, it is mandatory to record the pupil size in photopic, mesopic, and scotopic conditions, corneal topography and tomography with placido-based curvature topographic systems, pachymetry, biometry, wavefront aberrometry, evaluation of tear film, determination of ocular dominance, ocular motility, and specular microscopy [6–10]. In addition to standard corneal topography, evaluation of corneal biomechanics is a good clinical adjunct in process of detecting subclinical keratoconus among eyes clinically deemed to have seemingly normal topography. Next to standard topography, corneal biomechanics analysis, as at the Oculus CORVIS tonometer, is gradually being introduced into practice today [11, 12]. Newer models of high-resolution swept-source OCT (SS-OCT) have been generating corneal epithelial thickness maps with standard anterior segment metrics, which is going to play a role in planning keratorefractive surgery and identification of early keratoconus [13]. Currently, modern wavefront aberrometers are incorporating corneal topography systems to calculate the contribution of corneal aberrations (anterior and posterior), and internal aberration (from the crystalline lens) to complete ocular wavefront. Therefore, taking into account the available data, clinicians are able to decide on the type of personalized (customized) ablation profiles [14, 15]. In cataract surgery or CLE/RLE candidates, besides standard preoperative assessment, IOL power calculation is crucial data for ensuring an effective surgery result. Calculation formulas are undergoing continuous improvements, with the latest formulas having shown promising precision and less refractive surprises [16]. As previously mentioned, machine learning technologies could create classification models using algorithms trained from data for achieving better results. One of the examples that are already present in clinical practice is the Kane formula [17].

It is also important to discuss the reasons for undergoing refractive surgery to identify patients with unrealistic expectations. It is extremely important to explain to patients that refractive procedures primarily serve to reduce spectacle independence in everyday situations.

2.2 Keratorefractive surgery

2.2.1 History of keratorefractive surgery

The beginnings of refractive surgery date back to ancient times. The first written records of cataract surgery date back to ancient Egypt in the fifth century BC [18]. The development of modern refractive surgery began in the mid-twentieth century. Tsutomu Sato introduced anterior and posterior keratotomy into clinical practice, and in 1939 published his results [19, 20]. The method is being further developed by Russian scientists Beliaev, Durnev, Yenaliev, and Fyodorov, who eventually introduced the radial keratotomy procedure to correct myopia [21–24]. Later on, José Barraquer in Colombia started developing the idea of lamellar corneal surgery to change the shape of the cornea. The idea arose from the observation that lamellar keratoplasty leads to a reduction in the cone in patients with keratoconus, and consequently to a reduction in myopia. In 1964, Barraquer described the principles of lamellar corneal surgery and called the procedure "keratomileusis," which means the formation of the cornea [25–27]. The development of excimer lasers began in the 1970s with experiments on a combination of rare gases (such as argon and xenon) and halogen gases (such as fluorine and chlorine) used as laser media. Trokel and Srinivasan were the first to suggest that an excimer laser could have unique qualities for performing corneal surgery. In 1983, they suggested that such a laser could be used to remove tissue lamellae to change the curvature of the cornea and make precise incisions in the cornea [28, 29]. Theo Seiler was the first person to use an excimer laser on the human eye. In 1985 he performed astigmatic keratotomy, and in 1986 he performed the first phototherapeutic keratectomy (PTK) [30–32]. Munnerlyn et al. developed a computer-generated algorithm that links the diameter of the treatment zone to the depth of ablation to induce a specific diopter change in the cornea. An algorithm known as the Munnerlyn formula was used to develop laser patterns for inducing specific changes in corneal curvature to achieve the desired diopter change [33]. Laser *in situ* keratomileusis (LASIK) is a modification of Barraquer's keratomileusis and automated lamellar keratoplasty [34, 35]. The first method was developed by Lucio Buratto and involved the creation of a corneal lenticule (free flap) with a microkeratome, then excimer laser ablation of the posterior surface of the cornea, and re-suturing of the corneal lenticule [36]. In the meantime, Ioannis Pallikaris was developing a method in another way. The method involved creating a lamellar corneal flap with a microkeratome of his design and using an excimer laser to remodel the remaining corneal stroma under the flap. Palikaris coined the term of the method "Laser *in situ* keratomileusis" (LASIK) [37, 38]. The first clinical femtosecond laser approved by the FDA for refractive surgery use was the IntraLase FS, launched in 2003 [39–41]. In 2007, new low pulse energy and high pulse frequency Fs laser was introduced by Ziemer – FEMTO LDV. Since 2009, versions of Fs laser systems for use in cataract surgery, such as the first LensX, have also begun to develop in practice [42]. The first clinical version of a lenticule extraction procedure was introduced in the clinical treatment of refractive surgery patients in 2007 [42] as "FLEx" (Femtosecond Lenticule Extraction). A refined surgical version, small-incision lenticule extraction (SMILE) was introduced by Carl Zeiss Meditec and in a short period has replaced FLEx in clinical use [43]. Currently, novel laser systems for SMILE procedure are introduced by ATOS from SCHWIND eye-tech solutions (SmartSight procedure) and ZIEMER LDV Z8 from Ziemer Ophthalmic Systems AG (CLEAR procedure, Corneal Lenticule Extraction for Advanced Refractive correction).

2.2.2 Photorefractive keratectomy (PRK)

Photorefractive keratectomy (PRK) involves the use of an excimer laser on the anterior surface of the cornea to change the refractive status of the eye by changing the curvature of the cornea [44–46]. Except for refractive purposes, excimer laser surface ablation is used in the treatment of corneal scars and dystrophies when it is called phototherapeutic keratectomy (PTK) [47]. PRK is considered the method of choice, both refractive and therapeutic, in patients with basal membrane dystrophy, given that postoperatively better epithelial adherence occurs [48]. It is indicated in myopia from 1.0 to 6.0D, hyperopia up to 3.0D, and astigmatism up to 6.0D. Treatment of higher corrections is not recommended due to the risk of postoperative corneal opacity [49]. The surgical technique involves removal of the epithelium by excimer laser (transepithelial PRK), knife, 18–20% ethanol alcohol, or sponge. After epithelial removal, excimer laser ablation is performed. After excimer laser ablation, 0.02% mitomycin C is optionally applied to prevent corneal clouding. Postoperative recovery includes postoperative discomfort caused by epithelial erosion and gradual recovery of visual acuity during epithelial healing (within 72 h).

2.2.3 Laser-assisted subepithelial keratectomy (LASEK/epi-LASIK)

LASEK was firstly performed by Dimitri Azar in 1996 and he called it PRK with "Alcohol assisted flap PRK" [50, 51]. The method was named LASEK by Massimo Camellin in 1999, who popularized the technique [52, 53]. The technique involves applying 20% ethanol to the epithelium for 30 seconds to weaken the hemidesmosomal connections between the epithelium and the Bowman's membrane, leading to the formation of an epithelial sheet that is easily removed before excimer laser ablation and repositioned at the original position. Epi-LASIK was described by Palikaris et al. [54]. The technique involves the use of an automated knife, similar to a microkeratome, to remove epithelium without the use of alcohol. Disadvantages of the method are the possibility of treating only myopia, and the inability to predict the level of postoperative pain and prolonged epithelial healing.

2.2.4 Laser in situ keratomileusis (LASIK)

Laser *in situ* keratomileusis (LASIK) is the most commonly performed surgical technique for the correction of most refractive errors [55, 56]. LASIK is performed in two steps and combines lamellar surgery with excimer laser application. The first step involves the formation of the anterior corneal flap, its lifting to expose the stroma of the cornea. Today, two technologies are available for flap formation—mechanical microkeratomes and femtosecond lasers, known as femtosecond LASIK (FsLASIK). The second step consists of applying an excimer laser to the stroma of the cornea to change the curvature of the corneal anterior surface. Upon completion of the excimer laser action, the flap is repositioned to its original position [37, 57, 58]. The advantages of LASIK over superficial ablations are the ability to treat a wider range of refractive errors, faster vision recovery, less postoperative discomfort, and lower incidence of postoperative corneal or scar fogging in higher refractive errors. The main disadvantages of the method are the complications related to the creation of the flap, and the risk of iatrogenic keratectasia [59–61].

2.2.5 Femtosecond refractive lenticule extraction (RELx) and small-incision lenticule extraction (SMILE)

Femtosecond refractive lenticular extraction (RELx) is a corneal refractive procedure based on intrastromal refractive lenticular extraction. In the RLEx procedure, the lenticule was accessed by creating a front corneal flap similar to the LASIK flap, while in the SMILE procedure, the lenticule, located under a 120–130 μm thick cap is accessed through a small 2–4 mm incision on the anterior surface of the cornea. The shape and size of the lenticule are based on a mathematical calculation for the correction of a specific refractive error, and the location and amount of tissue extracted are similar to that of LASIK. The advantages of the method are related to the absence of possible complications related to the formation of the flap, less impact on the biomechanical stability of the cornea, less pronounced dryness of the eye, and less induced aberrations of higher order. The main disadvantages of the method are the possibility of treating only myopia and lower amounts of astigmatism. In case of residual refractive error, currently, only a surface ablation procedure is advised for correction [62–65].

2.2.6 Multifocal laser ablation profiles

Multifocal laser ablations for the treatment of presbyopia are still in the developmental stage. The multifocal cornea produces a simultaneous image on the retina, and the brain selects the appropriate image depending on whether the person is looking into the distance or at close range while the other image remains blurred. Potential side effects of these procedures are dysphotopsia and monocular diplopia. In this type of ablation protocol, the laser is used to create a multifocal surface on the cornea (changing the strength of the refractive gradient over the pupil) to correct ametropia at a distance and near. A central hyper-positive zone is created for proximity correction, leaving the middle corneal periphery for distance correction. Since some studies reported an unacceptable rate of losing CDVA using this kind of protocol, the procedure did not get widespread clinical use [66–68]. In recent times, the correction of presbyopia aims the change corneal asphericity and thus, using spherical aberration, increasing the depth of focus. The protocol is called Laser Blended Vision (LBV) and currently has been reported far better tolerated than multifocal ablation procedures [69].

2.3 Corneal implants/inlays

Spectacle independence is all the more sought after, so new surgical treatments are being invented to provide glasses-free life. The idea of keratophakia brought new light to presbyopia treatment [70, 71]. One of the introduced treatments initiated by this idea was corneal inlays [72–75]. Raindrop is a corneal inlay shaped like a clear lenticule made of hydrogel, which is permeable to oxygen, fluids, and nutrients. The lens is 2 mm wide, 32 μm thick in the center with decreasing thickens to about 10 μm in the periphery, and has no refractive power; therefore, it induces hyperpolate corneal shape allowing good near and intermediate vision with negligibly affected distance vision. It is placed in the non-dominant eye under the corneal flap or intracorneal pocket at 120–200 μm depth at the center of the light constricted pupil [72–74]. Until 2017 around 4000–6000 Raindrops were implanted worldwide but in November 2018 the manufacturer asked for a device recall due to postoperative haze [76, 77]. Kamra inlay uses the pinhole principle to facilitate near vision. This opaque ring shaped inlay is made of polyvinylidene fluoride and carbon. It is 6 μm thick, 3.6 mm diameter wide with a central 1.6 mm aperture. The inlay is placed in the nondominant eye 250 μm deep into the lamellar corneal pocket. If LASIK is done earlier, the inlay is placed 100–110 μm below the corneal flap and centration is based on the first Purkinje image. Around 20,000 Kamra inlays have been implanted and generally, there was a high satisfaction rate with both distant and near vision [75, 78, 79].

Presbia Flexivue Microlens is a refractive corneal inlay with a plano central zone surrounded by rings of varying additional power between +1.25D and + 3.5D. It is 3 mm wide, 15–20 μm thick, and is made of hydroxyethyl methacrylate and methyl methacrylate. It is placed over the first Purkinje image in a femtosecond creating a corneal pocket that is 280–300 μm deep. The overall satisfaction among patients was high but between other inlays, UCDVA showed a significant decrease from preoperative to postoperative values, but no changes in binocular UCDVA [74, 75, 80–82]. Best indications for corneal inlays are phakic, presbyopic patients, 41 to 65 years of age, who have low manifest refraction, who do not require correction for clear distance vision, but who do require near correction [78, 83]. Inlays are also indicated as a therapeutic model in keratoconus eyes. One of the most used ones is the Intacs corneal implant by Additional Technology Inc. It consists of two segments designed to be placed in the periphery of the cornea, at approximately two-thirds depth, and are surgically inserted through a small radial incision in the corneal stroma [84, 85]. They are composed of two clear segments made from polymethylmethacrylate (PMMA), each having an arc length of 150°, and are available in six thicknesses—0.210, 0.250, 0.300, 0.350, 0.400 and 0.450 mm [86]. Aimed populations that can benefit from Intacs are patients with keratoconus older than 21 years of age who have progressive vision deterioration, clear corneas with at least 450 μm corneal tissue at the proposed incision site and transplantation as the only remaining treatment option. Contraindications for Intacs are corneas below 449 μm at the incision site, patients with autoimmune and immunodeficiency disorders, pregnant and nursing women, patients with recurrent corneal erosion and other corneal dystrophies, and patients taking isotretinoin or amiodarone hydrochloride [86, 87].

2.4 Phakic intraocular lenses (pIOLs)

Phakic intraocular lenses (pIOLs) are one of the available surgical option for the treatment of ametropia [88]. When the natural crystalline lens is clear and usually has retained its accommodative function pIOLs are used. They are an effective and relatively safe option for surgical treatment of refractive errors with a special emphasis on very high refractive errors in both myopic and hyperopic eyes [89]. It has been generally accepted that refractive surgery is an effective and safe way of treating refractive errors. The first choice for surgical treatment is the cornea, the ubiquitous and commoditized nature of excimer lasers today has popularized surgical options [90]. The issue is when a refractive surgeon is met with a challenge of very high prescriptions or other confounding factors, such as thin corneas, or other factors that increase the risk for an adverse outcome for corneal refractive surgery. The most commonly accepted range for laser vision correction in corneal refractive surgery is between 10 diopters of myopia to 5 diopters of hyperopia with up to 5 diopters of cylindrical correction. For patients with high motivation and a clear crystalline lens with no presbyopia, that fall outside these limits or have other factors connected to a potentially adverse outcome, phakic IOLs present a great option [89]. There are two refractive pIOLs approved for correcting refractive errors—anterior chamber and posterior chamber pIOLs [91].

2.4.1 Anterior chamber pIOLs

Anterior chamber pIOLs in use today are made by Ophtec, a Dutch company, their anterior chamber lens is called ArtiLens, there are two types—a flexible version ArtiFlex and a rigid PMMA version Artisan [92]. These lenses were at one time distributed by AMO, now Johnson & Johnson Vision, and many surgeons will use them under their old names Veriflex and Verisyse. The ArtiFlex is a foldable pIOL that is inserted through an opening of 3.2 mm, it is fixated on the iris using an enclavation technique, the powers range from −14.5 to −2.0, there is a toric version available with powers from −13.5 to −1.0 and cylinder ranging from −5.0 to −1.0. The Artisan is a rigid PMMA pIOL that has an optic diameter of 5 or 6 mm the powers available range from −15.5 to +12.0. These pIOLs are also fixated on the iris but as they are not foldable they require a larger incision either 5 or 6 mm depending on the optic diameter [92]. There was another option, Alcon CACHET, an angle-supported anterior chamber pIOL was an additional variant, but was discontinued during 2014 due to endothelial cell loss as a serious side effect. Endothelial cell loss occurs due to contact of endothelium layer and pIOL surface, causing corneal endothelial decompensation which leads to corneal edema (overhydration), and in the advanced stage, bullous keratopathy [93].

2.4.2 Posterior chamber pIOLs

Posterior chamber phakic IOLs are a different approach that wants to avoid endothelial cell loss by moving the pIOL behind the iris plane. But by moving the pIOL behind the iris and just above the crystalline lens, there are new potential issues that can arise. The first issue is angle closure glaucoma, as the pIOL can reduce the aqueous fluid outflow by pushing the iris angle, inducing very high IOP. Previous generations of pIOL designs required a small iridotomy creation to facilitate aqueous fluid outflow [94]. The second issue is that the pIOL could block the flow of fluid around the optic and into the anterior chamber, the iridotomy was also beneficial in these cases. The third issue was in case of pIOL touching the capsule of the crystalline lens, an early onset cataract can form [95]. The three big issues today are mostly avoided by the use of modern diagnostic tools and surgical experience. The new posterior chamber pIOLs have very strict sizing guides to adjust the size of the pIOL to the sulcus of the patient to avoid the lens closing the iridocorneal angle, proper sizing also ensures a large enough vault between the pIOL and crystalline lens, and the block of fluid flow is rectified by new pIOLs with a center hole for unobstructed flow [96]. Currently, there is only one generally adopted posterior chamber pIOL, STAAR Surgical Visian ICL. STAAR Surgical has patented the design and material of their lenses, these are very soft collamer-based pIOLs that are implanted with minimally invasive 3.2 mm injectors, and the folded lens is placed in the sulcus after it unfolds in the iris plane. Visian ICL comes in spherical powers from −18.0 to +10.0 diopters, and there is a toric variant from +0.5 to +6.0 diopters of the cylinder. The ICL is produced in four sizes, 12.1 mm, 12.6 mm, 13.2 mm, and 13.7 mm to fit the size of the sulcus of the patient as best as possible [92, 97]. STAAR Surgical Visian ICL is a great option for patients that are not suitable candidates for corneal refractive surgery and are not ready for refractive lens exchange due to their age.

2.5 Cataract surgery and refractive lens exchange

2.5.1 History of cataract surgery and evolution of intraocular lenses

The first records of cataract surgery date back to antiquity, where couching was the only method of resolving optical path opacity, but without replacing the refractive property (power) of the removed crystalline lens [18, 98]. At a later age, about 600 BC a primitive version of extracapsular cataract extraction was described by an Indian surgeon Sushruta [99]. It was not until the 18th century, in 1947, that the forerunner of modern cataract surgery—extracapsular cataract extraction (ECCE) was performed by Jacques Daviel [100, 101]. A few years later, in 1753 Samuel Sharp performed intracapsular cataract extraction (ICCE) [102]. During the next decade, ICCE was considered as a method of choice for cataract surgery. The main difficulties of these procedures were related to complications, such as high risks of postoperative infection, prolonged wound healing (10–12 mm), vitreous prolapse, and retinal ablation. In 1961 Tadeusz Krwawicz invented cryoextraction, a freezing method for removing the cataractous lens [103]. The introduction of phacoemulsification in 1967 by Dr. Charles Kelman was the basis and beginning of today's modern cataract surgery [104]. Concurrently, the idea of replacing the cataractous lens with artificial optics was developing, starting from Sir Harold Ridley who observed in the 2nd World War that one of the pilots had a plastic shrapnel eye injury, without causing foreign body reaction. Guided by that, he developed the first intraocular lens (IOL) made of polymethylmethacrylate (PMMA) for insertion in the eye after cataractous lens removal [105]. Various materials have been tried for IOLs, and finally in the late 1970s flexible, silicone lens was brought into use. The primary aim of introducing flexible IOLs was to avoid the disadvantages of PMMA, such as larger incisions and consequent postoperative astigmatism. Silicone IOLs rapidly adopted and conquered the market during the 1980s [106]. In 1989, the first commercially available three-piece silicone IOL was introduced (PhacoFlex SI-18 by AMO, now Johnson & Johnson Vision) [107]. Further on, in the 1980s, Barret developed the first hydrogel IOL made of soft hydrophilic material (IOGEL PC-12) implanted in 1983 [108]. Following closely, hydrophobic acrylic IOLs were developed, which represent the most common implanted foldable IOL today [109, 110]. The combination of innovations, such as the phacoemulsification technique, foldable IOL, and even the use of topical anesthesia [111], has ensured the development of modern cataract surgery. Over the next few decades, attempts were made to introduce lasers into ophthalmic surgery. Bille and Schanzlin were the first to propose ultrashort laser pulses for treating cataracts back in 1993 [112] and the first clinical results of femtosecond laser use in cataract surgery (Femtosecond-Laser-Assisted cataract surgery - FLACS) was reported by Nagy et al. [113]. In parallel with the development of surgical methods, the evolution of an IOL design has moved in the direction of correcting all working distances, trying to minimize or even remove spectacle independence [114]. With the introduction of multifocal lenses, an era began in which cataract surgery became refractive surgery. Since the 1980s, bifocal, trifocal, quadrifocal IOLs have been designed, and toric IOLs have been introduced to correct astigmatism [115]. As refractive surgery has developed widely, with increasing needs of working patients, occasional refractive surprises became a problem in clinical practice due to patient dissatisfaction. In this name, supplementary IOLs, such as SulcoFlex by Rayner, have been developed as one of the possible surgical correction options [116–119]. Accommodative IOL was developed to provide better distance corrected near visual acuity and higher levels of spectacle independence than standard monofocal IOLs but also producing minimal unwanted visual disturbances, such as halos and glares and contrast sensitivity compared with multifocal IOLs. The first accommodative FDA-approved IOL was CrystaLens by Bausch & Lomb Inc. [120, 121]. In an attempt of overcoming the drawbacks of multifocal and accommodative IOLs, EDOF design was developed, with the first FDA approval for Tecnis Symfony by Johnson & Johnson Vision [122]. The main principle of EDOF design is a single elongated focal point that enhances the depth of focus (range of vision), and therefore significantly reduces potential halos and glares induced by multifocal IOL by eliminating the overlapping of near and far images [123–125].

2.5.2 Monofocal intraocular lenses

Monofocal intraocular lenses are the most common type of IOL used in cataract surgery. They are designed to correct a patient's visual acuity for far distances, with the need for an optical aid for near vision. Lenses are usually indicated in patients with extremely high myopic or hyperopic refraction, amblyopia, macular degeneration, dry eye syndrome, history of previous ocular surgery, ocular trauma, autoimmune diseases, or connective tissue diseases.

Currently, monofocal IOLs are mainly represented as hydrophobic acrylic lenses with an aspheric surface design. Aspheric types of IOLs are eliminating positive spherical aberration of the prolate cornea, improving functional vision and reducing side effects, such as low contrast sensitivity or low night-driving performance. The functional benefit and optical advantages of aspheric IOL technology are related to pupil size, depth of focus, IOL centration, and customization. Since it is pupil-size dependent, some studies have shown that aspheric IOLs offer little or almost no benefit in smaller pupils [126–129]. Therefore, when it comes to customization, preoperative assessment is extremely important, which in addition to standard measurements includes corneal topographic analysis, and the values of corneal aberrations, especially spherical aberration. According to the obtained parameters, the final decision on the type of IOL is given.

2.5.3 Presbyopia-correcting intraocular lenses

With the development and increase in cataract surgical treatment, the patient's expectation regarding postoperative outcomes is also increasing, as they seek to achieve independence from spectacles and favorable visual outcomes at both near and far distances to meet the needs of everyday activities [130–132]. Nowadays, in a presbyopia-correcting pool of IOLs, multifocal and extended range of vision (EDOF) IOLs are most prevalent in clinical use. Multifocal IOLs in the initial variant had a diffractive design, and afterward, refractive design was introduced. Diffractive IOLs had one variant with or without apodization, where the central (near) area is surrounded by concentric rings with decreasing heights [133] and the second variant with an aspheric anterior surface and a posterior surface with diffractive rings [134, 135]. Refractive IOL design has an asymmetrical shape of the central (near) segment to provide a sort of transition between zones of IOL [136, 137]. Trifocal diffractive IOL was introduced to improve intermediate vision with a third focus, at 80 cm. The first one in clinical use was FineVision IOL by Physiol, further followed by At LISA tri by Zeiss, and RayOne Trifocal by Rayner. In comparison with a traditional trifocal IOL, quadrifocal IOL has three added powers for near and intermediate vision, providing more continuous vision. One example of IOL with quadrifocal design is PanOptix by Alcon, which uses a specific optical technology to redirect the focal point at 120 cm to the distance focal point for amplified performance [138].

After introducing a technology designed to improve the range of vision, especially at intermediate distances, EDOF IOLs gained high popularity in refractive cataract surgery. An EDOF technology development arose from the necessity to obviate drawbacks of monofocal and multifocal IOLs – providing better vision for intermediate distance without compromising functional vision, reducing contrast sensitivity, or inducing disturbances, such as halos and glares. Currently, there are four different EDOF technologies [139]—diffractive optics IOL (Tecnis Symfony and Synergy IOL, Tecnis Eyhance IOL by Johnson & Johnson Vision, and AT LARA by Zeiss- hybrid multifocals) [125, 140] non-diffractive optics IOL (AcrySof IQ Vivity IOL by Alcon and SiFI Mini WELL IOL by SIFI MedTech Srl.) [141, 142], small-aperture IOL (IC-8 IOL by AcuFocus Inc.) [143], and bioanalogic IOL (Wichterle IOL-Continuous Focus - WIOL-CF by Medicem) [144].

Conflict of interest

The authors declare no conflict of interest.

Acronyms and abbreviations

LASIK	laser in situ keratomileusis
SMILE	small-incision Lenticule extracton
IOL	intraocular lens
SS-OCT	swept-source optical coherence tomography
CLE	clear lens extraction
RLE	refractive lens exchange
PTK	photo therpeutic keratectomy
FLEx	femtosecond lenticule extraction
PRK	photo refractive keratectomy
LASEK	laser assisted sub-epithelial keratectomy
UCDVA	uncorrected distance visual acuity
PMMA	polymethyl methacrylate
PIOL	phakic intraocular lens
ECCE	extracapsular cataract extraction
ICE	intracapsular cataract extraction
FLACS	femtosecond laser assisted cataract surgery
EDOF	extended depth of focus

Author details

Maja Bohač* and Mateja Jagić
University Eye Hospital Svjetlost, Zagreb, Croatia

*Address all correspondence to: maja.bohac@svjetlost.hr

References

[1] Kim TI, Alio Del Barrio JL, Wilkins M, Cochener B, Ang M. Refractive surgery. Lancet. 2019;**393**:2085-2098

[2] Ang M, Mehta JS, Chan C, Htoon HM, Koh JC, Tan DT. Refractive lenticule extraction: Transition and comparison of 3 surgical techniques. Journal of Cataract and Refractive Surgery. 2014;**40**:1415-1424

[3] Arbelaez MC, Versaci F, Vestri G, Barboni P, Savini G. Use of a support vector machine for keratoconus and subclinical keratoconus detection by topographic and tomographic data. Ophthalmology. 2012;**119**:2231-2238

[4] Smadja D, Touboul D, Cohen A, Doveh E, Santhiago MR, Mello GR, et al. Detection of subclinical keratoconus using an automated decision tree classification. American Journal of Ophthalmology. 2013;**156**(237-46):e231

[5] Yousefi S, Yousefi E, Takahashi H, Hayashi T, Tampo H, Inoda S, et al. Keratoconus severity identification using unsupervised machine learning. PLoS One. 2018;**13**:e0205998

[6] Myung D, Schallhorn S, Manche EE. Pupil size and LASIK: A review. Journal of Refractive Surgery. 2013;**29**(11):734-741

[7] Rosen ES, Gore CL, Taylor D, Chitkara D, Howes F, Kowalewski E. Use of digital infrared pupilometer to assess patient suitability for refractive surgery. Journal of Cataract and Refractive Surgery. 2002;**28**(8):1433-1438

[8] Ambrosio R Jr, Alonso RS, Luz A, Cova Velarde LG. Corneal-thickness spatial profile and corneal-volume distribution: Tomographic indices to detect keratoconus. Journal of Cataract and Refractive Surgery. 2006;**32**(11):1851-1859

[9] Albietz JM, McLennan SG, Lenton LM. Ocular surface management of photorefractive keratectomy and laser in situ keratomileusis. Journal of Refractive Surgery. 2003;**19**(6):636-644

[10] Snir M, Kremer I, Weinberger D, Sherf I, Axer-Siegel R. Decompensation of exodeviation after corneal refractive surgery for moderate to high myopia. Ophthalmic Surgery, Lasers & Imaging. 2003;**34**(5):363-370

[11] Roberts CJ, Mahmoud AM, Bons JP, Hossain A, Elsheikh A, Vinciguerra R, et al. Introduction of two novel stiffness parameters and interpretation of air puff-induced biomechanical deformation parameters with a dynamic Scheimpflug analyzer. Journal of Refractive Surgery. 2017;**33**:266-273

[12] Ambrosio R Jr, Lopes BT, Faria-Correia F, Salomao MQ, Buhren J, Roberts CJ, et al. Integration of Scheimpflug-based corneal tomography and biomechanical assessments for enhancing ectasia detection. Journal of Refractive Surgery. 2017;**33**:434-443

[13] Ang M, Baskaran M, Werkmeister RM, Chua J, Schmidl D, Aranha Dos Santos V, et al. Anterior segment optical coherence tomography. Progress in Retinal and Eye Research. 2018;**66**:132-156

[14] Amigo A, Martinez-Sorribes P, Recuerda M. Refractive changes induced by spherical aberration in laser correction procedures: An adaptive optics study. Journal of Refractive Surgery. 2017;**33**:470-474

[15] Gatinel D, Malet J, Dumas L. Polynomial decomposition method

for ocular wavefront analysis. Journal of the Optical Society of America. A, Optics, Image Science, and Vision. 2018;**35**:2035-2045

[16] Shajari M, Kolb CM, Petermann K, Bohm M, Herzog M, de'Lorenzo N, et al. Comparison of 9 modern intraocular lens power calculation formulas for a quadrifocal intraocular lens. Journal of Cataract and Refractive Surgery 2018;44:942-948

[17] Connell BJ, Kane JX. Comparison of the Kane formula with existing formulas for intraocular lens power selection. BMJ Open Ophthalmology. 2019;**4**:e000251

[18] Ascaso F, Lizana J, Cristobal J. Cataract surgery in ancient Egypt. Journal of Cataract & Refractive Surgery. 2009;**35**(3):607-608. DOI: 10.1016/j.jcrs.2008.11.052

[19] Sato T. Treatment of conical cornea (incision of Descemet's membrane). Acta Soc Ophthalmol Jpn. 1939;**43**:544-555

[20] Sato T, Akiyama K, Shibata H. A new surgical approach to myopia. American Journal of Ophthalmology. 1953;**36**(61):823-829

[21] Yenaleyev FS. Experience in surgical treatment of myopia. Annals of Ophthalmology USSR. 1979;**3**:52-55

[22] Durnev VV. Characteristics of surgical correction of myopia after 16 and 32 peripheral anterior nonperforating incisions. In: Fyodorov SN, editor. Surgery for Anomalies in Ocular Refraction. Moscow: The Moscow Research Institute for Ocular Microsurgery; 1981. pp. 33-35

[23] Durnev VV, Ivanshina AA. Possibility of maximal elongation of incisions in radial keratotomy. In: Fyodorov SN, editor. Surgery for Anomalies in Ocular Refraction. Moscow: The Moscow Research Institute for Ocular Microsurgery; 1981. pp. 19-22

[24] Fyodorov SN, Agranovsky AA. Long-term results of anterior radial keratotomy. Journal of Ocular Pharmacology and Therapeutics. 1982;**1**:217-223

[25] Barraquer JI. Keratomileusis. International Surgery. 1967;**48**(2):103-117

[26] Barraquer JI. Keratomileusis for myopia and aphakia. Ophthalmology. 1981;**88**(8):701-708

[27] Barraquer JI. The history and evolution of keratomileusis. International Ophthalmology Clinics. 1996;**36**(4):1-7

[28] Srinivasan R. Kinetics of the ablative photodecomposition of organic polimers in the far ultraviolet (193 nm). Journal of Vacuum Science and Technology B. 1983;**1**(4):923-926

[29] Trokel SL, Srinivasan R, Braren B. Excimer laser surgery of the cornea. American Journal of Ophthalmology. 1983;**96**(6):710-715

[30] Seiler T, Wolensak J. In vivo experiments with the excimer laser technical parameters and healing process. Ophthalmologica. 1986;**192**(2):65-70

[31] Seiler T, Kahle G, Kriegerovski M. Excimer laser (193nm) myopic keratomileusis in sighted and blind human eyes. Refractive & Corneal Surgery. 1990;**6**(3):165-173

[32] Seiler T. Photorefractive keratectomy: European experience. In: Thompson FB, PJ MD, editors. Color Atlas/Text of Excimer Laser Surgery: The Cornea. New York: Igaku-Shoin; 1993. pp. 53-62

[33] Munnerlyn CR, Koons SJ, Marshall J. Photorefractive keratectomy: A technique for laser refractive surgery.

Journal of Cataract and Refractive Surgery. 1988;**14**(1):46-52

[34] RuizL, RowseyJ. Insitukeratomileusis. Investigative Ophthalmology & Visual Science. 1988;**29**:392

[35] Peyman GA. Method for modifying corneal curvature. US patent 4840175. 1989

[36] Buratto L, Ferrari M, Rama P. Excimer laser intrastromal keratomileusis. American Journal of Ophthalmology. 1992;**113**(3):291-295

[37] Pallikaris I, Papatsanaki M, Stathi E, Frenschock O, Georgiadis A. Laser in situ keratomileusis. Lasers in Surgery and Medicine. 1990;**10**(5):463-468

[38] Pallikaris I, Papatzanaki M, Siganos D, Tsilimbaris MK. A corneal flap technique for laser in situ keratomileusis. Human studies. Archives of Ophthalmology. 1991;**109**(12):1699-1702

[39] Ratkay-Traub I, Juhasz T, Horvath C, Suarez C, Kiss K, Ferincz I, et al. Ultra-short pulse (femtosecond) laser surgery: Initial use in LASIK flap creation. Ophthalmology Clinics of North America. 2001;**14**:347-355

[40] Kezirian GM, Stonecipher KG. Comparison of the IntraLase femtosecond laser and mechanical keratomes for laser in situ keratomileusis. Journal of Cataract and Refractive Surgery. 2004;**30**:804-811

[41] Lubatschowski H, Maatz G, Heisterkamp A, Hetzel U, Drommer W, Welling H, et al. Application of ultrashort laser pulses for intrastromal refractive surgery. Graefe's Archive for Clinical and Experimental Ophthalmology. 2000;**238**:33-39

[42] Nagy ZZ, McAlinden C. Femtosecond laser cataract surgery. Eye and Vision. 2015;**2**:1-8

[43] Wei S, Wang Y. Comparison of corneal sensitivity between FS-LASIK and femtosecond lenticule extraction (ReLEx flex) or small-incision lenticule extraction (ReLEx smile) for myopic eyes. Graefe's Archive for Clinical and Experimental Ophthalmology. 2013;**251**:1645-1654

[44] Puliafito CA, Steinert RF, Deutsch TF, Hillenkamp F, Dehm EJ, Adler CM. Excimer laser ablation of the cornea and lens: Experimental studies. Ophthalmology. 1985;**92**(6):741-748

[45] Gartry DS, Kerr Muir MG, Marshal J. Excimer laser photorefractive keratectomy: 18 month follow up. Ophthalmology. 1992;**99**(8):1209-1219

[46] Campos M, Nielsen S, Szerenyi K, Garbus JJ, McDonnell PJ. Clinical follow-up of phototherapeutic keratectomy for treatment of corneal opacities. American Journal of Ophthalmology. 1993;**115**(4):433-440

[47] Sher NA, Bowers RA, Zabel RW, i sur. Clinical use of 193nm excimer laser int he treatment of corneal scars. Archives of Ophthalmology. 1991;**109**(4):491-498

[48] Örndahl MJ, Fagerholm PP. Phototerapeutic keratectomy for map-dot-fingerprint corneal dystrophy. Cornea. 1998;**17**(6):595-599

[49] Lee YG, Chen WY, Petrol WM, Cavanagh HD, Jester JV. Corneal haze after photorefractive keratectomy using different epithelial removal techniques: Mechanical debridement versus laser scrape. Ophthalmology. 2001;**108**(1):112-120

[50] Azar DT, Taneri S. LASEK. In: Azar DT, editor. Refractive Surgery. 2nd ed. Philadelphia: Elsevier Inc; 2007. pp. 239-247

[51] Azar DT, Ang RT, Lee JB. Laser subepithelial keratomileusis: electron microscopy and visual outcomes of flap photorefractive keratectomy. Current Opinion in Ophthalmology. 2001;**12**(4):323-328

[52] Camellin M. Laser epithelial keratomileusis for myopia. Journal of Refractive Surgery. 2003;**19**(6):666-670

[53] Cimberle M, Camellin M. LASEK may offer the advantages of both LASIK and PRK. Ocular Surgery News. International Edition. 1999;**10**:28

[54] Pallikaris IG, Naoumidi II, Kalyvianaki MI, Katsanevaki VJ. Epi LASIK: Comparative histological evaluation of mechanical and alcohol-assisted epithelial separation. Journal of Cataract and Refractive Surgery. 2003;**29**(8):1496-1501

[55] Duffey RJ, Learning D. US trends in refractive surgery. 2003 ISRS/AAO survey. Journal of Refractive Surgery. 2005;**21**(1):87-91

[56] Schmack I, Auffarth GU, Epstein D, Holzer MP. Refractive surgery trends and practice style in Germany over a 3 year period. Journal of Refractive Surgery. 2010;**26**(3):202-208

[57] Gatinel D. LASIK for myopia, hyperopia and astigmatism. In: Azar DT, editor. Refractive Surgery. 2nd ed. Philadelphia: Elsevier Inc; 2007. pp. 165-182

[58] Carr JD, Stulting RD, Thompson KP, Waring GO 3rd. Laser in situ keratomileusis: surgical technique. Ophthalmology Clinics of North America. 2001;**14**(2):285-294

[59] Moshirfar M, Gardiner JP, Schliesser JA, i sur. Laser in situ keratomileusis flap complications using mechanical microkeratome versus femtosecond laser: Retrospective comparison. Journal of Cataract and Refractive Surgery. 2010;**36**(11):1925-1933

[60] Twa MD, Nichols JJ, Joslin CE. Characteristics of corneal ectasia after LASIK for myopia. Cornea. 2004;**23**(5):447-457

[61] Ou RJ, Shaw EL, Glasgow BJ. Keratectasia after laser in situ keratomileusis (LASIK): Evaluation of the calculated residual stromal bed thickness. American Journal of Ophthalmology. 2002;**134**(5):771-773

[62] Reinstein DZ, Carp GI, Archer TJ, Gobbe M. Outcomes of small incision Lenticule extraction (SMILE) in low myopia. Journal of Refractive Surgery. 2014;**30**(12):812-818

[63] Blum M, Kunert K, Schroder M, Sekundo W. Femtosecond lenticule extraction for the correction of myopia: Preliminary 6-month results. Graefe's Archive for Clinical and Experimental Ophthalmology. 2010;**248**(7): 1019-1027

[64] Shah R, Shah S, Sengupta S. Results of small incision lenticule extraction: All-in-one femtosecond laser refractive surgery. Journal of Cataract and Refractive Surgery. 2011;**37**(1):127-137

[65] Pedersen IB, Bak-Nielsen S, Vestergaard AH, Ivarsen A, Hjortdal J. Corneal biomechanical properties after LASIK, ReLEx flex, and ReLEx SMILE by Scheimpflug-based dynamic tonometry. Graefe's Archive for Clinical and Experimental Ophthalmology. 2014;**252**(8):1329-1335

[66] Jung WS, Kim MJ, Park SH, Joo C. Multifocal corneal ablation for hyperopic presbyopes. Journal of Refractive Surgery. 2008;**24**(9):903-910

[67] Alarcón A, Anera RG, Soler M, Del Barco LJ. Visual evaluation of different multifocal corneal models for the correction of presbyopia by laser ablation. Journal of Refractive Surgery. 2011;**27**(11):833-836

[68] El Danasoury AM, Gamaly TO, Hantera M. Multizone LASIK with peripheral near zone for correction of presbyopia in myopic and hyperopic eyes: 1-year results. Journal of Refractive Surgery. 2009;**25**(3):296-230

[69] Reinstein DZ, Archer TJ, Gobbe M. Laser blended vision for presbyopia correction. In: Pallikaris IG, Plainis S, Charman WN, editors. Presbyopia: Origins, Effects and Treatment. Thorofare, NJ: SLACK Incorporated; 2012

[70] Barraquer JI. Modification of refraction by means of intracorneal inclusions. International Ophthalmology Clinics. 1966;**6**:53-78

[71] Barraquer JI. Keratophakia. Transactions of the ophthalmological societies of the United Kingdom. 1972;**92**:499-516

[72] Lindstrom RL, Macrae SM, Pepose JS, Hoopes PC Sr. Corneal inlays for presbyopia correction. Current Opinion in Ophthalmology. 2013;**24**:281-287

[73] Konstantopoulos A, Mehta JS. Surgical compensation of presbyopia with corneal inlays. Expert Review of Medical Devices. 2015;**12**:341-352

[74] Arlt E, Krall E, Moussa S, Grabner G, Dexl A. Implantable inlay devices for presbyopia: The evidence to date. Clinical Ophthalmology. 2015;**9**:129-137

[75] Moarefi MA, Bafna S, Wiley W. A review of presbyopia treatment with corneal inlays. Ophthalmology and Therapy. 2017;**6**(1):55-65. DOI: 10.1007/s40123-017-0085-7

[76] Yoo A, Kim JY, Kim MJ, Tchah H. Hydrogel inlay for presbyopia: Objective and subjective visual outcomes. Journal of Refractive Surgery. 2015;**31**:454-460

[77] FDA Class 1 recall of Raindrop Near Vision Inlay, (initiated Nov 2018; Create Mar 2019, Available from: https://www.accessdata.fda.gov/scripts/cdrh/cfdocs/cfRes/res.cfm?ID=169984

[78] Acu Focus Inc. KAMRA Inlay, Informational Manual for Professional Use. CA, USA: U.S. Food and Drug Administration; 2015. Available from: https://www.accessdata.fda.gov/cdrh_docs/pdf12/p120023d.pdf

[79] Vukich JA, Durrie DS, Pepose JS, Thompson V, van de Pol C, Lin L. Evaluation of the small-aperture intracorneal inlay: Three year results from the cohort of the U.S. Food and Drug Administration clinical trial. Journal of Cataract and Refractive Surgery. 2018;**44**:541-556

[80] Malandrini A, Martone G, Menabuoni L, Catanese AM, Tosi GM, Balestrazzi A, et al. Bifocal refractive corneal inlay implantation to improve near vision in emmetropic presbyopic patients. Journal of Cataract and Refractive Surgery. 2015;**41**:1962-1972

[81] Limnopoulou AN, Bouzoukis DI, Kymionis GD, Panagopoulou SI, Plainis S, Pallikaris AI, et al. Visual outcomes and safety of a refractive corneal inlay for presbyopia using femtosecond laser. Journal of Refractive Surgery. 2013;**29**:12-18

[82] Baily C, Kohnen T, O'Keefe M. Preloaded refractive-addition corneal inlay to compensate for presbyopia

implanted using a femtosecond laser: One-year visual outcomes and safety. Journal of Cataract and Refractive Surgery. 2014;**40**:1341-1348

[83] ReVision Optics Inc. Raindrop near Vision Inlay, Information Manual for Professional Silver Spring, Maryland, USA: U.S. Food and Drug Administration; 2016. Available from: https://www.accessdata.fda.gov/cdrh_docs/pdf15/p150034c.pdf

[84] Vega-Estrada A, Alio JL. The use of intracorneal ring segments in keratoconus. Eye and Vision. 2016;**3**:8

[85] Vega-Estrada A, Alio JL, Brenner LF, Javaloy J, Plaza Puche AB, Barraquer RI, et al. Outcome analysis of intracorneal ring segments for the treatment of keratoconus based on visual, refractive, and aberrometric impairment. American Journal of Ophthalmology. 2013;**155**: 575-84.e571

[86] Additional Technology Inc. (2004) Intrastromal Corneal Ring Segment, INTACS: Information Manual for Professional Use. Silver Spring, Maryland, USA: U.S. Food and Drug Administration; Available from: https://www.accessdata.fda.gov/cdrh_docs/pdf4/h040002c.pdf

[87] Warrak EL, Serhan HA, Ayash JG, et al. Long-term follow up of intracorneal ring segment implantation in 932 keratoconus eyes. Journal Français d'Ophtalmologie. 2020;**43**(10):1020-1024

[88] Kohnen T, Shajari M. Phake Intraokularlinsen [Phakic intraocular lenses]. Der Ophthalmologe. 2016;**113**(6):529-538. German. DOI: 10.1007/s00347-016-0283-z

[89] Nanavaty MA, Daya SM. Refractive lens exchange versus phakic intraocular lenses. Current Opinion in Ophthalmology. 2012;**23**:54-61

[90] Sugar A, Rapuano CJ, Culbertson WW, Huang D, Varley GA, Agapitos PJ, et al. Laser in situ keratomileusis for myopia and astigmatism: Safety and efficacy: A report by the American Academy of ophthalmology. Ophthalmology. 2002;**109**:175-187

[91] Ang M, Gatinel D, Reinstein DZ, Mertens E, Alió Del Barrio JL, Alió JL. Refractive surgery beyond 2020. Eye (London, England). 2021;**35**(2):362-382. DOI: 10.1038/s41433-020-1096-5

[92] Hou C, Li H, Li J, Li J, Peng H, Wang Q. Artisan versus Artiflex phakic intraocular lens implantation in the treatment of moderate to high myopia: meta-analysis. BMC Ophthalmology. 2021;**21**(1):171. DOI: 10.1186/s12886-021-01930-6

[93] Galvis V, Villamil JF, Acuña MF, Camacho PA, Merayo-Lloves J, Tello A, et al. Long-term endothelial cell loss with the iris-claw intraocular phakic lenses (artisan®). Graefe's Archive for Clinical and Experimental Ophthalmology. 2019;**257**(12):2775-2787. DOI: 10.1007/s00417-019-04506-9

[94] Pop M, Payette Y. Refractive lens exchange versus iris-claw artisan phakic intraocular lens for hyperopia. Journal of Refractive Surgery. 2004;**20**:20-24

[95] Gonvers M, Bornet C, Othenin-Girard P. Implantable contact lens for moderate to high myopia: Relationship of vaulting to cataract formation. Journal of Cataract and Refractive Surgery. 2003;**29**:918-924

[96] Barsam A, Allan BD. Excimer laser refractive surgery versus phakic intraocular lenses for the correction of moderate to high myopia. Cochrane Database of Systematic Reviews. 2014;**6**:CD007679. DOI: 10.1002/14651858.CD007679.pub4

[97] Shen Y, Wang L, Jian W, Shang J, Wang X, Ju L, et al. Big-data and artificial-intelligence-assisted vault prediction and EVO-ICL size selection for myopia correction. The British Journal of Ophthalmology. 2021:bjophthalmol-2021-319618. DOI: 10.1136/bjophthalmol-2021-319618 [Online ahead of print]

[98] Feigenbaum A. Early history of cataract and the ancient operation for cataract. American Journal of Ophthalmology. 1960;**49**:305-326

[99] Grzybowski A, Ascaso FJ. Sushruta in 600 B.C. introduced extraocular expulsion of lens material. Acta Ophthalmologica. 2014;**92**(2):194-197. DOI: 10.1111/aos.1203

[100] Rucker CW. Cataract: A historical perspective. Investigative Ophthalmology. 1965;**4**:377-383

[101] Davis G. The evolution of cataract surgery. Missouri Medicine. 2016;**113**(1):58-62

[102] Hubbell AA. Samuel sharp, the first surgeon to make the corneal incision in cataract extraction with a single knife: A biographical and historical sketch. Medical Library and Historical Journal. 1904;**2**(4):1-268

[103] Nagy ZZ. History of cataract surgery from ancient times to today. Developments in Health Sciences. 2020;**2**(4):88-92. DOI: 10.1556/2066.2019.00002 [Accessed: March 12, 2022]

[104] Kelman CD. Phaco-emulsification and aspiration. A new technique of cataract removal. A preliminary report. American Journal of Ophthalmology. 1967;**64**(1):23-35

[105] Apple DJ, Sims J. Harold Ridley and the invention of the intraocular lens. Survey of Ophthalmology. 1996;**40**(4):279-292. DOI: 10.1016/s0039-6257(96)82003-0

[106] Obstbaum SA. Development of foldable IOL materials. Journal of Cataract and Refractive Surgery. 1995;**21**(3):233. DOI: 10.1016/s0886-3350(13)80119-8

[107] Steinert RF, Bayliss B, Brint SF, Giamporcaro JE, Hunkeler JD. Long-term clinical results of AMO PhacoFlex model SI-18 intraocular lens implantation. Journal of Cataract and Refractive Surgery. 1995;**21**(3):331-338. DOI: 10.1016/s0886-3350(13)80143-5

[108] Barrett GD, Constable IJ, Stewart AD. Clinical results of hydrogel lens implantation. Journal of Cataract and Refractive Surgery. 1986;**12**(6):623-631. DOI: 10.1016/s0886-3350(86)80076-1

[109] Cionni RJ. Intraocular lenses to restore and preserve vision following cataract surgery. In: Kohnen T, Koch DD, editors. Cataract and Refractive Surgery. Essentials in Ophthalmology. Berlin, Heidelberg: Springer; 2006. DOI: 10.1007/3-540-30796-6_1

[110] Werner L. Biocompatibility of intraocular lens materials. Current Opinion in Ophthalmology. 2008;**19**(1):41-49. DOI: 10.1097/ICU.0b013e3282f20132

[111] Fichman RA. Use of topical anesthesia alone in cataract surgery. Journal of Cataract and Refractive Surgery. 1996;**22**(5):612-614. DOI: 10.1016/s0886-3350(96)80019-8

[112] Bille JF, Schanzlin D. Method for Removing Cataractous Material. US Patent US5246435A, 1993

[113] Nagy Z, Takacs A, Filkorn T, Sarayba M. Initial clinical evaluation

of an intraocular femtosecond laser in cataract surgery. Journal of Refractive Surgery. 2009;**25**:1053-1060

[114] Gale RP, Saldana M, Johnston RL, Zuberbuhler B, McKibbin M. Benchmark standards for refractive outcomes after NHS cataract surgery. Eye (London, England). 2009;**23**(1):149-152. DOI: 10.1038/sj.eye.6702954

[115] Werner L. Intraocular lens evolution in the past 25 years as told by the journal of Cataract & Refractive Surgery. Journal of Cataract and Refractive Surgery. 2021;**47**(2):147-149. DOI: 10.1097/j.jcrs.0000000000000558

[116] Gundersen KG, Makari S, Ostenstad S, Potvin R. Retreatments after multifocal intraocular lens implantation: An analysis. Clinical Ophthalmology. 2016;**10**:365-371

[117] Makhotkina NY, Dugrain V, Purchase D, Berendschot T, Nuijts R. Effect of supplementary implantation of a sulcus-fxated intraocular lens in patients with negative dysphotopsia. Journal of Cataract and Refractive Surgery. 2018;**44**(2):209-218

[118] Makhotkina NY, Berendschot TT, Beckers HJ, Nuijts RM. Treatment of negative dysphotopsia with supplementary implantation of a sulcus-fixated intraocular lens. Graefe's Archive for Clinical and Experimental Ophthalmology. 2015;**253**(6):973-977 82 T.C.Y. Chan et al

[119] Falzon K, Stewart OG. Correction of undesirable pseudophakic refractive error with the Sulcofex intraocular lens. Journal of Refractive Surgery. 2012;**28**(9):614-619

[120] Zhou H, Zhu C, Xu W, Zhou F. The efficacy of accommodative versus monofocal intraocular lenses for cataract patients: A systematic review and meta-analysis. Medicine. 2018;**97**(40):e12693

[121] Alio JL, Alio Del Barrio JL, Vega-Estrada A. Accommodative intraocular lenses: Where are we and where we are going. Eye and Vision. 2017;**4**:16. DOI: 10.1186/s40662-017-0077-7

[122] FDA News Release. http://www.fda.gov/NewsEvents/Newsroom/PressAnnouncements/ucm511446.htm [Accessed: March 11, 2022]

[123] Akella SS, Juthani VV. Extended depth of focus intraocular lenses for presbyopia. Current Opinion in Ophthalmology. 2018;**29**(4):318-322

[124] Gallego AA, Bara S, Jaroszewicz Z, Kolodziejczyk A. Visual Strehl performance of IOL designs with extended depth of focus. Optometry and Vision Science. 2012;**89**(12):1702-1707

[125] Cochener B, Concerto Study G. Clinical outcomes of a new extended range of vision intraocular lens: International Multicenter concerto study. Journal of Cataract and Refractive Surgery. 2016;**42**(9):1268-1275

[126] Sandoval HP, Fernández de Castro LE, Vroman DT, Solomon KD. Comparison of visual outcomes, photopic contrast sensitivity, wavefront analysis, and patient satisfaction following cataract extraction and IOL implantation: Aspheric vs spherical acrylic lenses. Eye (London, England). 2008;**22**(12):1469-1475. DOI: 10.1038/sj.eye.6702925

[127] Rocha KM, Soriano ES, Chalita MR, Yamada AC, Bottos K, Bottos J, et al. Wavefront analysis and contrast sensitivity of aspheric and spherical intraocular lenses: A randomized prospective study. American Journal of Ophthalmology. 2006;**142**:750-756

[128] Rocha KM, Soriano ES, Chamon W, Chalita MR, Nosé W. Spherical aberration and depth of focus in eyes implanted with aspheric and spherical intraocular lenses: A prospective randomized study. Ophthalmology. 2007;**114**(11):2050-2054. DOI: 10.1016/j.ophtha.2007.01.024

[129] Werner L, Olson RJ, Mamalis N. New technology IOL optics. Ophthalmology Clinics of North America. 2006;**19**:469-483

[130] Du W, Lou W, Wu Q. Personalized aspheric intraocular lens implantation based on corneal spherical aberration: A review. International Journal of Ophthalmology. 2019;**12**(11):1788-1792. DOI: 10.18240/ijo.2019.11.19

[131] Braga-Mele R, Chang D, Dewey S, et al. ASCRS cataract clinical committee multifocal intraocular lenses: Relative indications and contraindications for implantation. Journal of Cataract and Refractive Surgery. 2014;**40**(2):313-322

[132] Schmickler S, Bautista CP, Goes F, Shah S, Wolffsohn JS. Clinical evaluation of a multifocal aspheric diffractive intraocular lens. The British Journal of Ophthalmology. 2013;**97**(12):1560-1564

[133] Lichtinger A, Rootman DS. Intraocular lenses for presbyopia correction: Past, present, and future. Current Opinion in Ophthalmology. 2012;**23**:40-46

[134] Montes-Mico R, Ferrer-Blasco T, Charman WN, Cervino A, Alfonso JF, Fernandez-Vega L. Optical quality of the eye after lens replacement with a pseudoaccommodating intraocular lens. Journal of Cataract and Refractive Surgery. 2008;**34**:763-768

[135] Kohnen T, Allen D, Boureau C, Dublineau P, Hartmann C, Mehdorn E, et al. European multicenter study of the AcrySof ReSTOR apodized diffractive intraocular lens. Ophthalmology. 2006;**113**:578-584

[136] Alio JL, Pinero DP, Plaza-Puche AB, Chan MJ. Visual outcomes and optical performance of a monofocal intraocular lens and a new-generation multifocal intraocular lens. Journal of Cataract and Refractive Surgery. 2011;**37**:241-250

[137] Rosen E, Alio JL, Dick HB, Dell S, Slade S. Efficacy and safety of multifocal intraocular lenses following cataract and refractive lens exchange: Metaanalysis of peer-reviewed publications. Journal of Cataract and Refractive Surgery. 2016;**42**:310-328

[138] Sudhir RR, Dey A, Bhattacharrya S, Bahulayan A. AcrySof IQ PanOptix intraocular Lens versus extended depth of focus intraocular Lens and trifocal intraocular Lens: A clinical overview. Asia-Pacific Journal of Ophthalmology (Phila). 2019;**8**(4):335-349. DOI: 10.1097/APO.0000000000000253

[139] Kohnen T, Suryakumar R. Extended depth-of-focus technology in intraocular lenses. Journal of Cataract and Refractive Surgery. 2020;**46**(2):298-304. DOI: 10.1097/j.jcrs.0000000000000109

[140] Kohnen T, Böhm M, Hemkeppler E, Schönbrunn S, DeLorenzo N, Petermann K, et al. Visual performance of an extended depth of focus intraocular lens for treatment selection. Eye. 2019;**33**:1556-1563

[141] Bellucci R, Curatolo MC. A new extended depth of focus intraocular lens based on spherical aberration. Journal of Refractive Surgery. 2017;**33**(389-394):13

[142] Savini G, Balducci N, Carbonara C, et al. Functional assessment of a new extended depth-of-focus intraocular lens. Eye (London, England). 2019;**33**(3):404-410. DOI: 10.1038/s41433-018-0221-1

[143] Dick HB, Elling M, Schultz T. Binocular and monocular implantation

of small aperture intraocular lenses in cataract surgery. Journal of Refractive Surgery. 2018;**34**:629-631

[144] Studeny P, Krizova D, Urminsky J. Clinical experience with the WIOL-CF accommodative bioanalogic intraocular lens: Czech National Observational Registry. European Journal of Ophthalmology. 2016;**26**:230-235

Section 2

Refractive Error

Chapter 2

Myopia

Pavol Vesely and Kamila Kopalova

Abstract

Short-sightedness -myopia-, is the most common refractive error in the world. The number of myopic people is rising worldwide. It causes range from those that are genetically determined to those influenced by the external environment. Several risks factors have been described that increase the likelihood of an increase in myopia. Manifestations of myopia in the eye vary, but they affect almost the entire eyeball; whether it's the cornea, the anterior chamber, or the posterior segment of the eye. It is on the posterior segment that damage to the intraocular tissues can occur, which seriously endangers visual functions. Therefore, the prevention of myopia plays an important role in stabilizing and limiting its growth.

Keywords: myopia, axial length, retinal pigment epithelium defects, lacquer cracks, chorioretinal atrophy, myopic cone, myopic chorioretinal atrophy, myopic maculopathy, peripheral myopic degeneration, prevention

1. Introduction

Myopia (short-sightedness) is the most common refractive error of the eye, in which the rays of light refracted by the lens converge at a point in front of the retina, so there is no sharp image on the retina. Its manifestation is poor visibility of distant objects. To correct the blurred image created on the retina in the short-sighted eye, it is necessary to reduce the refractive power of the cornea, the lens, or both, so that the light rays converge more posteriorly to create a sharp image on the retina. Because the cornea represents approximately two-thirds of the total refractive power of the eye, in refractive surgery we try to increase its radius and reduce its thickness to correct myopia. Other options are correction with negative lenses in glasses or intraocular lens implantation.

In myopia, the distance from the nodal point (optic center) to the retina is greater than is found in an emmetropic eye, and therefore, the projected image will be larger than normal, unlike in those with hypertropia, in whom the refractive apparatus projects a smaller image [1].

According to the main cause, we divide myopia into axial, refractive and mixed. In axial myopia, the main cause is an increase in the axial (anteroposterior) length of the eye. The average axial length of the eye in the Caucasian population is 23.33 mm [2]. Within the average range of axial length, an increase in axial length by 1mm corresponds to a decrease of approximately 3 diopters in glasses.

In refractive myopia, the optical refractive power of the cornea and/or the lens is increased. It could be caused by a decreased radius of optical surfaces (e.g., keratoconus, lenticonus). An increase in the refractive indices of the lens, such as that which occurs in nuclear cataract, could also cause refractive myopia. The mixed type of myopia occurs when both of the aforementioned causes are present together.

Based on the amount of myopia (the value of refraction in diopters), we can categorise light (up to -3 D), medium (up to -6 D) and high myopia (over -6 D).

In general, we classify myopia into two groups: non-pathological and pathological myopia. Non-pathological myopia is also commonly referred to as simple or school myopia. Simple myopia is usually up to -6D where the structures of the eye develop within normal limits without signs of degeneration of the sclera, retina or choroid which are typical of pathological myopia.

Pathological myopia (PM), also known as degenerative or malignant myopia, is characterised by a refractive error of at least -6 D, an axial length of more than 26.5 mm, and degenerative changes affecting the sclera, choroid and retina. These changes are concentrated in the areas from the ora serrata to the equator zone and at the posterior pole of the eye [3].

2. Prevalence

Myopia is a major global public health and socio-economic problem, the incidence of which has risen sharply around the world in recent decades [4]. Myopia is usually an underestimated eye disease. Although impaired vision due to myopia can often be corrected with visual aids such as glasses, contact lenses, or refractive surgery, uncorrected refractive error is still the leading cause of visual impairment worldwide, accounting for at least 33% of visual impairments [5–7]. A total of 153 million people over the age of 5 years are estimated to be visually impaired due to uncorrected myopia and other refractive errors, of which eight million will become blind. The incidence of myopia is increasing from west to east [8]. In the Central European Caucasian population, the prevalence of myopia is estimated at 23% [9], and in the young Asian population, it is up to 80-90% [10].

High myopia is associated with a risk of irreversible visual impairment and blindness due to higher risks of macular and retinal complications. Holden et al. showed that 25% of all myopic subjects would eventually develop pathological myopia and 50% of those with pathological myopia would have poorer vision until late adulthood [11]. Pathological myopia is one of the leading causes of vision loss in developed countries, especially in the younger population (in those younger than 50 years old). Older generations have shorter eyes on average relative to younger adults [2]. When comparing pathological myopia, adolescents and children have a significantly lower prevalence compared to adults. This supports the idea that myopic macular changes are time-dependent because of mechanical retinal tension caused by axial extension of the eye. It has been found that myopic changes of the macula and optic disc are commonly found in highly myopic eyes in young adults [12]. It is therefore likely that the disease burden of pathological myopia will increase in the future due to high myopia. The aging effect seen in myopia will contribute to this process [4].

According to a global prediction for 2050, the incidence of pathological myopia may increase to more than 200 million in the future [11]. Studies have reported that pathological myopia is a major cause of blindness or visual impairment in 7% of the Western population and 12-27% of the Asian population [4].

3. Biometric and anatomical changes

3.1 Biometric changes

Most cases of myopia are strongly related to increased axial length. Increased axial length may cause changes in many other biometrical parameters. These changes could be the result of proportional adjustment during emmetropisation or simply a result of an increase in anatomical space.

Opinions on corneal changes in myopia are controversial. Several analyses revealed only a weak correlation between increasing corneal refractive power (steeper radius of curvature) and increasing degree of myopia, while others do not indicate any correlation or opposite relationship [2]. Long-term studies suggest that changes in corneal curvature during childhood and early adulthood are minimal and unrelated to the extent of myopia progression. Although corneal thickness does not change with refractive error, a decrease in corneal hysteresis (an estimate of corneal biomechanical strength or viscoelasticity) has been observed with an increase in the degree of myopia in children and adults [4, 13].

Changes in the depth of the anterior chamber in childhood are indirectly related to changes in the thickness of the lens (the thinner the lens, the deeper the anterior chamber). The anterior chamber is usually deeper in myopes compared to emmetropes, whilst, conversely, the lens is thinner in myopes [14].

In contrast to the anterior segment, changes in the posterior segment (especially the vitreous, choroid and sclera) are more pronounced in myopes compared to non-myopic eyes. The axial length, or more precisely the depth of the vitreous cavity, is the primary biometric contributor to the refractive error. The axial length of the eyeball and the depth of the vitreous cavity increases in emmetropic children by approximately 0.16 mm per year from 6 to 10 years of age, decelerating to 0.05 mm per year from 11 to 14 years [15]. In short-sighted children aged 6 to 11 years (corrected by spectacles or contact lenses), average growth rates of approximately 0.30 mm per year have been reported, with larger vitreous cavities and axial elongations observed in younger women with myopic parents [16]. The extent of myopia correction slows the rate of eye growth and the progression of myopia during childhood, in some cases by up to 50% [4].

3.2 Choroid

The choroid supplies oxygen and nutrients to the outer layers of the retina, and also regulates intraocular pressure and eye temperature. High myopia is associated with profound changes in the choroid. In the process of myopization, the eye elongates but does not form additional tissue, therefore, the sclera, choroid and retina are stretched and thinned. The choroid thickness differs from normal at extreme axial lengths (extremely short and long) [17]. The choroid thickness decreases with increasing myopia and axial length in both adults and children. The most pronounced thinning is in the foveal area compared to non-myopic subjects [18]. Significant choroidal thinning is observed in high myopia and in eyes with posterior staphyloma and may contribute to atrophy and myopic maculopathy. Areas of completely missing choroidal vessels could be found in very high myopes. Myopic maculopathies are a variety of lesions, all of which involve vascular changes, namely diffuse chorioretinal atrophy, irregular chorioretinal atrophy, macular atrophy, lacquer cracks, and myopic choroidal neovascularization [4].

A colour Doppler ultrasonographic study showed that choroidal circulation was reduced in highly myopic eyes due to its marked thinning [19]. Because the choroid supplies oxygen and nutrition to the retinal pigment epithelial cells (RPE) and outer layers of the retina, impaired choroidal circulation may be partly responsible for retinal dysfunction associated with vision loss [20].

The reduction in choroid thickness occurs with age in both non-myopes and myopes. In the elderly, the choroid may also show reduced thickness in a process known as age-related choroidal atrophy (ARCA) [21]. These patients have a normal axial length but show tessellation of the fundus and peripapillary atrophy of the beta zone, much the same as older high myopes. Eyes with reduced choroid thickness as part of ARCA are more likely to have pseudodrusen, whilst highly myopic eyes almost never have pseudodrusen. Based on studies, ARCA was defined as a reduction in choroidal thickness due to age of less than 125 μm [20].

3.3 Sclera

Anatomical changes occurring in the collagen fibers of the sclera contribute to the axial elongation of the eye, as well as the formation and progression of staphyloma. Scleral thinning associated with axial myopia is primarily limited to the posterior pole of the eye due to the redistribution of scleral tissue. Myopia causes several changes in the composition of the sclera. There is a general loss of collagen and proteoglycans. At the onset of myopia, the ongoing synthesis of type I collagen is decreased, and existing collagens and proteoglycans are degraded by matrix metalloproteinases [20].

Scleral thinning around the optic nerve head makes myopic eyes more susceptible to glaucoma damage. Histological studies have shown that scleral thinning associated with axial length elongation is most pronounced near the posterior pole, while scleral thickness anterior to the equator does not differ significantly between eyes of different axial lengths [22]. Slight anterior scleral thinning occurs during accommodation, especially in myopic eyes, probably due to the biomechanical forces of the ciliary muscle [23].

3.4 Retina

Retinal changes in myopia are closely related to the changes in the sclera and choroid. RPE cells are flatter and larger, and in some places, pigment cells and photoreceptors are replaced by Müller cells. The Bruch membrane shows various changes, including thinning and ruptures.

4. Complications

In summary, anatomical changes occurring during myopia are:

- increasing axial length, anterior chamber depth and vitreous cavity depth
- decreasing retinal, choroidal and scleral thickness
- the vessels of the retina, choroid, ciliary body narrow and lengthen
- there is mechanical tension and focal ruptures of the Bruch's membrane-RPE-choriocapillaris complex
- increase in lamina cribrosa defects around the optic nerve head.

These changes can lead to complications associated either with high or pathological myopia. Most typical are those related to the posterior pole of the eye because of the prolongation of the axial length and thus the stretching of the posterior pole and the formation of staphyloma. Scleral ectasia affecting the posterior pole of the eye is relatively common and usually leads to a poor visual prognosis. Most complications associated with myopic maculopathy can lead to irreversible damage to photoreceptors, leading to decreased central visual acuity [24].

4.1 Posterior staphyloma

The presence of posterior staphyloma is the most characteristic finding of pathological myopia. A staphyloma is a circumscribed bulging of the scleral wall that has a radius of curvature smaller than the surrounding curvature of the eyewall. A primary (simple) staphyloma is an area that has only one radius of curvature. Combined staphyloma consist of two or more staphyloma.

Posterior staphyloma is characterised by the presence of a sudden sharply demarcated margin. Compared to the normal retina, the bulged area is relatively pale and is associated with increased visibility of choroidal vessels. Staphyloma depth correlates with the extent of scleral thinning. Posterior staphyloma is often associated with chorioretinal atrophy. In fact, these two symptoms are the most common macular finding associated with myopia, occurring in approximately 20-23% of highly myopic eyes in adults [24]. Increasing age and axial length are relevant risk factors associated with the occurrence of pathological changes in highly myopic patients, as well as with the occurrence of staphyloma. The posterior staphyloma deepens with age, changes its shape, and thus increases the number of combined staphyloma. The prevalence of posterior staphyloma increases with age; it occurs in 53.5% of highly myopic patients aged 60-86 years [24].

The first classification of posterior staphyloma was suggested by Curtin in 1977 [25]. Ohno-Matsui modified and simplified the classical Curtin classification. The new classification stratifies posterior staphyloma into 6 types according to their location and extent [26].

Due to the extreme thinning of the choroid in highly myopic eyes, the curvatures of both the retina and Bruch's membrane closely mimic the curvature of the sclera. However, this is not the case with emmetropic eyes, because the choroid is much thicker [26]. Many authors have evaluated the role of staphyloma in the development of chorioretinal atrophy. Clinical quantification of posterior staphyloma showed that shorter staphyloma depth was associated with poorer best-corrected visual acuity and a higher occurrence of myopic choroidal neovascularization. On the other hand, larger staphyloma has been associated with a higher prevalence of cone formation, RPE defects, lacquer cracks, and chorioretinal atrophy [27].

4.2 Tilted disc syndrome

With an inferior staphyloma, the nerve is usually at the border of the staphyloma and has an inclined appearance. This appearance is called tilted optic disk syndrome. Tilted disc syndrome (TDS), also known as Fuch's Coloboma, is a congenital anomaly that occurs in up to 3.5% of the population [28]. It is an abnormality consisting of inferonasal tilting of the optic disc. It may cause superior bitemporal visual field defects. These defects could be confused with chiasmal lesions; however, the visual field defects in TDS can cross the vertical meridian. Other types of defects in TDS include altitudinal or arcuate defects. They may be confused with glaucomatous changes.

4.3 Myopic cone

A myopic cone is one of the first signs to develop on the posterior pole in myopic eyes. It has the appearance of a pale and sharply demarcated crescent-shaped area. This is the area of the translucent sclera which is created by the pulling and thinning of the retina and choroid from the optic nerve. It tends to increase with increasing myopia and axial length. Myopic cone and tessellated fundus are the earliest lesions that develop in eyes with pathological myopia, and these lesions can also be seen in children and young individuals. A myopic cone without the occurrence of other pathologies has no effect on visual acuity.

4.4 Myopic maculopathy

Myopic maculopathy is described by a simplified and systematic classification based on a meta-analysis of pathological myopia (META-PM) [29]. Myopic maculopathy lesions have been categorized into five categories from 0 to 4: 0. no myopic retinal lesions; 1. tessellated fundus; 2. diffuse chorioretinal atrophy; 3. patchy chorioretinal atrophy and 4. macular atrophy. Two additional categories were added to them and were included as 'plus signs': lacquer cracks and myopic choroidal neovascularization (CNV). Fuchs' spots were categorized under the term myopic CNV. The reason for the separate listing of additional lesions ("plus signs") is that they are associated with central vision loss, however, they do not fall into any main category, and they may develop or coexist with any of the categories of myopic maculopathy described above.

Myopic choroidal neovascularisation is a vision-threatening complication in many ocular diseases, including pathological myopia [30]. Pathological myopia is the most common cause of CNV in people under the age of 50 and is the second most common cause of CNV after age-related macular degeneration (AMD) [4]. Approximately 5-11% of patients with pathological myopia develop CNV, usually type 2 [4, 31].

Lacquer cracks are spontaneous cracks in Bruch's membrane-RPE-choriocapillaris complex. After the spontaneous resorption of subretinal hemorrhages caused by these ruptures, we can observe lacquer cracks in the corresponding area of previous bleeding. They appear clinically as fine, linear, irregular, yellowish subretinal lines at the posterior pole of highly myopic eyes. They occur most frequently in the macular area.

In highly myopic eyes, atrophy of the retinal pigment epithelium may occur. It is assumed that the pathophysiology is similar to age-related choroidal atrophy [20]. This fundoscopic finding is described as tessellated fundus. It has no effect on central visual acuity.

Diffuse chorioretinal atrophy appears as a vaguely demarcated yellowish lesion on the posterior pole of the eye in highly myopic patients. It begins to appear around the optic disc and spreads to the entire macular area. Its incidence increases with age as well as with increased axial length. It begins to appear around the age of 40 [32].

Patchy chorioretinal atrophy appears as a gray-white, clearly demarcated lesion in the macular area or around the optic disc. It is characterized by complete atrophy of the RPE, choroid and outer layers of the retina. It has a characteristic white colour because the sclera is visible through the transparent retinal tissue. With increasing age, areas of irregular atrophy enlarge and cluster with each other. Patchy chorioretinal atrophy causes the formation of absolute scotomas. Extra-foveal patches rarely involve the fovea and central visual acuity is spared [20].

In macular atrophy, progressive choroidal atrophy is followed by loss of retinal pigment epithelium and outer retinal layers. These areas of atrophy eventually merge to form large geographical areas of atrophy. Macular atrophy is similar to patchy chorioretinal atrophy, but is cantered on the fovea, which significantly impairs the central vision.

4.5 Dome-shaped macula

The dome-shaped macula (DSM) is an anterior bulging of the macula of >50μm above the level of the outer RPE line on the posterior staphyloma associated with high myopia and a posterior staphyloma. It can be visualized by OCT [33]. Several theories have been proposed, but the exact pathophysiology of DSM remains unclear. It was thought to be either due to coarsening of the choroid, collapse of the posterior wall of the eye, or vitreomacular traction. More recent evidence suggests that it seems to be related to a localized scleral thickening. The presence of DSM is associated with an increased risk of complications. Eyes with complications have a thinner choroid, thicker sclera, and higher dome height [33]. Complications include serous retinal detachment, CNV, epiretinal membrane, lamellar and full-thickness macular hole, and foveal or extra-foveal retinoschisis.

4.6 Myopic traction maculopathy

In 2014, Panozzo and Mercanti introduced the term myopic traction maculopathy (MTM) to describe the spectrum of foveal traction changes in highly myopic eyes. MTM included the following alterations: foveoschisis/maculoschisis/retinoschisis (FS/MS/RS), retinal/foveal detachment (RD/FD), lamellar macular holes (LMH) and full-thickness macular holes (FTMH) with (MHRD) or without RD [34].

The presence of posterior staphyloma in highly myopic patients plays a key role in the subsequent development of MTM, as the elasticity of the retina cannot compensate for the posterior scleral bulging. This rigidity of the retina can be caused by many factors, including vascular rigidity, the presence of epiretinal membrane (ERM), vitreomacular traction syndrome (VMTS), cortical vitreous remnants, or incomplete posterior vitreous detachment. The internal limiting membrane (ILM) could also be thickened or stiffened [20, 35].

Myopic foveoschisis (FS) can be diagnosed ophthalmoscopically in some cases, but OCT examination is necessary to make a correct diagnosis and to monitor development. Myopic foveoschisis involves the gradual separation of the retinal layers, which remain joined by Müller cells [20]. Several classifications have been proposed for FS. Some are based on the location or amount of its extension. Others are based on the involvement of different retinal layers [35]. Most patients with FS may be relatively asymptomatic, especially when the eyes do not develop more serious complications, such as a macular hole. FS can last for many years without significantly affecting vision. Some patients complain of metamorphopsia before a decrease in visual acuity. Regular OCT examination should be performed in highly myopic eyes with posterior staphyloma. For eyes with stable disease, observation is a sufficient approach.

The progression of FS can lead to complications, including foveal detachment, lamellar macular holes (LMH) and full-thickness macular holes. LMH is a common finding on OCT in asymptomatic myopic patients. Surgery is only necessary for the presence of clear vitreous traction or decreased visual acuity. Epiretinal proliferation associated with myopic LMH tends to be more prevalent and is more adherent to the posterior hyaloid than in non-myopic eyes [36]. Some authors perform fovea-sparing ILM peeling to protect the fovea. This approach is helpful in myopic FS with vitreomacular traction, where forces exerted during the peeling could damage weakened fovea and lead to FTHM [37].

The development of FTMH in myopic eyes is associated with significant visual impairment. Anteroposterior and tangential traction of the vitreous on the macula is closely related to the development of MH. In the presence of posterior staphyloma, which promotes retinal layer cleavage, myopic MH is commonly associated with FS, which is an important difference compared to emmetropic MH. Overall, the presence of concomitant FS indicates a worse anatomical and functional prognosis, which may even lead to retinal detachment.

The goal of surgical treatment is complete closure of FTHM, as well as to maintain or improve visual acuity. The gold standard of treatment is posterior vitrectomy, posterior hyaloid dissection, and ILM peeling. It is important to remove the entire vitreous from the macular surface. Vitreoschisis is common in myopic patients. ILM peeling in highly myopic eyes is a demanding surgical manoeuvre due to several factors, including greater axial length, retinal thinning, weak staining of ILM and difficulty identifying the exact location of the MH. Many surgeons perform a full ILM peeling across the macula to the vascular arcades in an effort to maximize the relief of tangential tractions. Several alternative techniques have been proposed to achieve a successful closure, especially in FTMH with FS. One of these techniques is the inverted ILM flap method [38]. This technique has several modifications where the ILM layer is placed inside or above the MH bed to anatomically close the macular hole [39]. At the end of surgery, it is important to perform the fluid-air exchange to prevent the ILM flap from slippage. Macular buckling surgery is another method of treating MTM. It relieves anterior-posterior traction by placing a buckle under the posterior pole and pushing it anteriorly. It could be made more effective by combination with pars plana vitrectomy [40].

4.7 Peripheral retinal degenerations

The main peripheral retinal degeneration changes associated with pathological myopia are lattice degenerations, white with/without pressure, pigment degenerations, paving stone degeneration and retinal holes. Each of these degenerations has its distinct morphology and prevalence, which varies with age and axial length. The dynamic interaction between the vitreous and the retina plays an important role in the development, appearance, and progression of these peripheral retinal degenerations. The combination of abnormal vitreoretinal adhesions, posterior vitreous traction, and vitreous liquefaction can lead to rhegmatogenous retinal detachment in highly myopic eyes. Early detection of peripheral retinal changes associated with high myopia through careful ophthalmoscopic examination or examination with a wide-angle viewing system is very important in preventing the most dangerous complication of peripheral degeneration—retinal detachment. Paving stone degeneration or pigment degeneration is considered a benign lesion without an increased risk of complications. Lattice or snail track degenerations are the most dangerous in terms of vitreoretinal adhesions, tear creation and subsequent rhegmatogenous retinal detachment. The most common peripheral degeneration in myopic adults and children is lattice degeneration [41, 42]. Whether or when to treat lattice degeneration in adult eyes has been a source of controversy. Prophylactic treatment for asymptomatic peripheral retinal degenerations in adults is not recommended [42, 43]. There is not sufficient data to strongly support prophylactic treatment of asymptomatic lesions [43]. However, treatment of lattice in the other eye of patients with rhegmatogenous retinal detachment reduces the risk of retinal detachment in the second eye from 5.1% to 1.8%. In addition, prophylactic treatment did not reduce the risk of detachment in the higher risk eyes with high myopia or extensive lattice [44]. Laser photocoagulation is the most common procedure in prophylactic treatment of peripheral degenerations. Buckles or encircling bands are sometimes used for prophylaxis.

4.8 Myopic optic neuropathy and glaucoma

Axial myopization leads to significant changes in the optic nerve head: enlargement of all three layers of the optic disc (Bruch membrane, choroidal and scleral orifice of the optic disc); enlargement and fusion of excavation; lengthening and thinning of the lamina cribrosa, peripapillary sclera and choroid, and rotation of the optic disc around the vertical axis. These changes, among others, such as the loss of the neuroretinal rim margin and thinning of the retinal nerve fiber layer (RNFL), make it difficult to distinguish between myopic changes and glaucoma-related changes. At the same time, these changes may make optic nerve head more vulnerable, which could explain the increased prevalence of glaucomatous optic neuropathy in highly myopic eyes [4]. Myopia is a risk factor for glaucoma. Eyes with high myopia had a sixfold increased risk of having primary open-angle glaucoma [45]. Highly myopic glaucoma eyes may have significantly lower IOP thresholds for optic nerve damage [4]. These factors make myopic glaucoma hard to diagnose and treat.

5. Risk factors

Myopia is a complex multifactorial disorder affected by genetic and environmental factors. Although genetic factors are the strongest influence, exposure to the environment plays an important role. Environmental factors can include occupational activities, work on computer displays and other light-emitting devices (electron microscopes, photographic equipment, lasers, etc.), stress and eye strain [20, 46].

Another explanation for the different perspectives on the role of genetic factors in myopia is the sensitivity of the human eye to very small changes in its anatomical structure. Small deviations from the normal structure could cause significant refractive errors. This is the reason why it is difficult to determine strength of the influence for specific genetic or environmental factors.

Genes in the proximity of loci associated with refractive error play different functions, including as neurotransmitters (GJD2, RASGRF1, GRIA4, etc.), involvement in retinoic acid metabolism (RDH5, RGR, RORB), and ion channel activity (KCNQ5, KCNJ2, KCNMA1, CACNA1D), or are involved in ocular and central nervous system development (SIX6, CHD7, ZIC2, and PRSS56). Although their individual effect is small, the overall effect of these genes may be highly coordinated [47]. Other genes associated with myopia encode extracellular matrix-related proteins (COL1A1, COL2A1 and MMP1, MMP2, MMP3, MMP9, MMP10) [4]. The PAX6 gene has a suggestive association with high myopia [48]. Any of these genes could cause a disruption in the balance between growth of the eye and emmetropization.

6. Prevention

The relationship between time outdoors and myopia onset has been documented in several epidemiologic studies [49]. A randomized trial of 952 schoolchildren in China showed that an intervention of 40 minutes per day spent outdoors decreased myopia onset by 9% after 3 years [50]. In animal studies, experiments in chicken and non-human primate animal models have shown that high illuminance levels of light (>15,000 Lux) can slow or even stop the development of experimentally induced myopia [49]. However, this amount of illuminance might be retinotoxic in the long term [51]. To achieve healthy exposure to daylight, an effort should be made to increase children's time spent outdoors with physical activity. These measurements could not only slow down myopia but increased physical activity could prevent obesity and its own health-related complications.

There are many other possible interventions to reduce the progression of myopia. In terms of refraction, atropine, pirenzepine and progressive addition spectacle lenses were effective. For axial length, atropine, orthokeratology, peripheral defocus modifying contact lenses, pirenzepine, and progressive addition spectacle lenses were effective. The most effective interventions are muscarinic antagonists, such as atropine and pirenzepine [52]. All used doses (high-dose (1% and 0.5%), moderate-dose (0.1%) and low-dose of (0.01%)) of atropine are effective [52]. High doses induce clinical symptoms such as changes in pupil size and accommodation and displayed a rapid rebound effect with myopia when the treatment was stopped [53]. On the other hand, low-dose atropine (0.01%) does not show the same rebound effect seen in higher doses and has fewer visual side effects [49]. The ATOM2 clinical trial showed that over 5 years, atropine 0.01% eye drops were more effective in slowing myopia progression with fewer visual side effects compared to higher doses of atropine. Furthermore, atropine 0.01% also caused minimal pupil dilation (0.8 mm), minimal loss of accommodation (2-3 D), and no near visual loss compared with higher doses [54].

Another way to prevent the progression of myopia is contact lenses with added myopic defocus. These lenses are bifocal soft contact lenses with a series of alternating defocusing and correction zones. The correcting zones match the distant prescription, while the defocusing zones have myopic defocus. Myopia progressed 25% slower in children in the bifocal lens group compared with those in the control group with single-vision soft contact lenses [55]. In another study, they achieved greater control in myopia progression (59%) and axial elongation (52%) with bifocals relative to single-vision 1-day contact lenses [56]. However, the quality of vision offered by these lenses may be reduced due to their myopic defocus which may result in poorer compliance [49].

Orthokeratology (OK) is a clinical technique to flatten the central cornea moderately while steepening the peripheral cornea using contact lenses (CLs) worn overnight [49]. OK lenses showed moderate effects on the change in axial length (AL) compared with single-vision spectacle lenses/placebo over a year [52]. The OK technique is less popular, probably due to the frequent discomfort of wearing lenses overnight and the risk of infectious keratitis. There is no relevant data on rebound effects of this method.

The therapeutic effect of bifocal or other types of multifocal spectacles on myopia progression has been evaluated in several trials. The correction of Myopia Evaluation Trial 2 (COMET 2) showed that the progressive-addition lenses used in this study were found to have a statistically but not clinically significant effect of slowing myopia progression in children with high accommodative lag and near esophoria [57]. A trial with bifocals, without and with prism, showed that both bifocal groups had less axial elongation (0.25 mm and 0.28 mm, respectively) than the single-vision lens group. It suggested that prismatic bifocals are more effective for myopic children with insufficient accommodation [58].

Myopia is a significant public health challenge, particularly in the urban environments of Asian countries. Whilst novel methods are emerging to control the progression of myopia, their principles are still unclear. A combination of these methods could yield a cumulative effect. Further studies are needed to confirm these assumptions.

Acknowlegments

Supported by grant KEGA 023 STU-4/2020.

Author details

Pavol Vesely* and Kamila Kopalova
Vesely Eye Clinic, Bratislava, Slovakia

*Address all correspondence to: palo.vesely@veselyok.com

References

[1] Yanoff M, Duker JS. Ophthalmology E-Book. Elsevier Health Sciences. Amsterdam, Netherlands: Elsevier B.V. (Corporate Office); 2018

[2] Popov I et al. Analysis of biometric parameters of 2340 eyes measured with optical biometer Lenstar LS900 in a Caucasian population. European Journal of Ophthalmology. 2022;**32**(1):213-220

[3] Wilkinson CP, Hinton DR, Sadda SR, Wiedemann P. Ryan's Retina E-Book. Elsevier Health Sciences. Netherlands, Amsterdam: Elsevier B.V. (Corporate Office); 2017

[4] Ang M, Wong TY. Updates on myopia: A clinical perspective. London, UK: Springer Nature; 2020. p. 305

[5] Popov I, Popova V, Sekac J, Krasnik V. Does every calculation formula fit for all types of intraocular lenses? Optimization of constants for tecnis ZA9003 and ZCB00 is necessary. Medicina (Mex.). 2021;**57**(4):319

[6] Sherwin JC et al. Uncorrected refractive error in older British adults: The EPIC-Norfolk Eye Study. The British Journal of Ophthalmology. 2012;**96**:991-996

[7] Popov I, Valašková J, Krásnik V, Tomčíková D. Effect of multiple variables on the refractive error after cataract surgery. Ceska Slov. Oftalmol. Cas. Ceske Oftalmol. Spolecnosti Slov. Oftalmol. Spolecnosti. 2019;**74**:158-161

[8] Resnikoff S, Pascolini D, Mariotti SP, Pokharel GP. Global magnitude of visual impairment caused by uncorrected refractive errors in 2004. Bulletin of the World Health Organization. 2008;**86**: 63-70

[9] Popov I, Valašková J, Štefaničková J, Krásnik V. Prevalence of refractive errors in the Slovak population calculated using the Gullstrand schematic eye model. Ceska Slov. Oftalmol. Cas. Ceske Oftalmol. Spolecnosti Slov. Oftalmol. Spolecnosti. 2017;**73**:113-117

[10] Wu P-C, Huang H-M, Yu H-J, Fang P-C, Chen C-T. Epidemiology of Myopia. Asia-Pacific Journal of Ophthalmology. 2016;**5**:386-393

[11] Holden BA et al. Global prevalence of myopia and high myopia and temporal trends from 2000 through 2050. Ophthalmology. 2016;**123**:1036-1042

[12] Koh V et al. Myopic maculopathy and optic disc changes in highly myopic young asian eyes and impact on visual acuity. American Journal of Ophthalmology. 2016;**164**:69-79

[13] Huang Y et al. Corneal biomechanics, refractive error, and axial length in Chinese primary school children. Investigative Ophthalmology & Visual Science. 2011;**52**:4923-4928

[14] Shih Y-F, Chiang T-H, Lin LL-K. Lens thickness changes among schoolchildren in Taiwan. Investigative Ophthalmology & Visual Science. 2009;**50**:2637-2644

[15] Zadnik K et al. Normal eye growth in emmetropic schoolchildren. Optometry Vision Science Official Publication of American Academy of Optometry. 2004;**81**:819-828

[16] Saw SM et al. Eye growth changes in myopic children in Singapore. The British Journal of Ophthalmology. 2005;**89**:1489-1494

[17] Popov I, Popova V, Krasnik V. Comparing the results of vitrectomy and sclerectomy in a patient with

nanophthalmic uveal effusion syndrome. Medicina (Mex.). 2021;**57**(120)

[18] Xiong S et al. Choroidal thickness in 3001 Chinese children aged 6 to 19 years using swept-source OCT. Scientific Reports. 2017;7:45059

[19] Akyol N, Kükner AS, Ozdemir T, Esmerligil S. Choroidal and retinal blood flow changes in degenerative myopia. Canadian Journal of Ophthalmology. 1996;**31**:113-119

[20] Ohno-Matsui K, Wu PC, Yamashiro K, Vutipongsatorn K, Fang Y, Cheung CMG, et al. IMI pathologic myopia. Investigative Ophthalmology & Visual Science. 2021;**62**(5):5-5

[21] Spaide RF. Age-related choroidal atrophy. American Journal of Ophthalmology. 2009;**147**:801-810

[22] Jonas JB, Ohno-Matsui K, Panda-Jonas S. Myopia: Anatomic changes and consequences for its etiology. Asia-Pacific Journal of Ophthalmology. 2019;**8**:355-359

[23] Consejo A, Radhakrishnan H, Iskander DR. Scleral changes with accommodation. Ophthalmic & Physiologic Optics: The Journal of the British College of Ophthalmic Opticians Optometry. 2017;**37**:263-274

[24] Ruiz-Medrano J et al. Myopic maculopathy: Current status and proposal for a new classification and grading system (ATN). Progress in Retinal and Eye Research. 2019;**69**:80-115

[25] Curtin BJ. The posterior staphyloma of pathologic myopia. Transactions of the American Ophthalmological Society. 1977;**75**:67-86

[26] Ohno-Matsui K. Proposed classification of posterior staphylomas based on analyses of eye shape by three-dimensional magnetic resonance imaging and wide-field fundus imaging. Ophthalmology. 2014;**121**:1798-1809

[27] Steidl SM, Pruett RC. Macular complications associated with posterior staphyloma. American Journal of Ophthalmology. 1997;**123**:181-187

[28] Kim YC, Moon J-S, Park H-YL, Park CK. Three dimensional evaluation of posterior pole and optic nerve head in tilted disc. Scientific Reports. 2018;**8**:1121

[29] Ohno-Matsui K et al. International photographic classification and grading system for myopic maculopathy. American Journal of Ophthalmology. 2015;**159**:877-883

[30] Horkovicova K, Popov I, Tomcikova D, Popova V, Krasnik V. The natural history of retinal vascular changes from infancy to adulthood in Wyburn-Mason Syndrome. Medicina (Kaunas, Lithuania). 2020;**56**:E598

[31] Wong TY, Ferreira A, Hughes R, Carter G, Mitchell P. Epidemiology and disease burden of pathologic myopia and myopic choroidal neovascularization: An evidence-based systematic review. American Journal of Ophthalmology. 2014;**157**:9-25

[32] Tokoro T. Atlas of Posterior Fundus Changes in Pathologic Myopia. Japan: Springer; 1998

[33] Jain M, Gopal L, Padhi TR. Dome-shaped maculopathy: A review. Eye. 2021;**35**:2458-2467

[34] Panozzo G, Mercanti A. Optical coherence tomography findings in myopic traction maculopathy. Archives of Ophthalmology. 2004;**1960**(122): 1455-1460

[35] Frisina R et al. Myopic traction maculopathy: Diagnostic and management strategies. Clinical Ophthalmology. 2020;**14**:3699-3708

[36] Lai T-T, Yang C-M. Lamellar hole-associated epiretinal proliferation in lamellar macular hole and full-thickness macular hole in high myopia. Retina. 2018;**38**:1316-1323

[37] Shimada N, Sugamoto Y, Ogawa M, Takase H, Ohno-Matsui K. Fovea-sparing internal limiting membrane peeling for myopic traction maculopathy. American Journal of Ophthalmology. 2012;**154**:693-701

[38] Hu X-T, Pan Q-T, Zheng J-W, Zhang Z-D. Foveal microstructure and visual outcomes of myopic macular hole surgery with or without the inverted internal limiting membrane flap technique. The British Journal of Ophthalmology. 2019;**103**:1495-1502

[39] Hirata A, Mine K, Hayashi K. Contractility of temporal inverted internal limiting membrane flap after vitrectomy for macular hole. Scientific Reports. 2021;**11**:20035

[40] Susvar P, Sood G. Current concepts of macular buckle in myopic traction maculopathy. Indian Journal of Ophthalmology. 2018;**66**:1772-1784

[41] Chen DZ et al. Peripheral retinal changes in highly myopic young Asian eyes. Acta Ophthalmology. 2018;**96**:e846-e851

[42] Bansal AS, Hubbard GB. Peripheral retinal findings in highly myopic children ≤10 years of age. Retina. 2010;**30**:S15-S19

[43] Wilkinson CP. Evidence-based analysis of prophylactic treatment of asymptomatic retinal breaks and lattice degeneration. Ophthalmology. 2000;**107**:12-15

[44] Folk JC, Arrindell EL, Klugman MR. The fellow eye of patients with phakic lattice retinal detachment. Ophthalmology. 1989;**96**:72-79

[45] Pan C-W et al. Differential associations of myopia with major age-related eye diseases: The Singapore Indian eye study. Ophthalmology. 2013;**120**:284-291

[46] Huang H-M, Chang DS-T, Wu P-C. The Association between near work activities and myopia in children—A systematic review and meta-analysis. PLoS One. 2015;**10**:e0140419

[47] Hysi PG, Wojciechowski R, Rahi JS, Hammond CJ. Genome-wide association studies of refractive error and myopia, lessons learned, and implications for the future. Investigative Ophthalmology & Visual Science. 2014;**55**:3344-3351

[48] Tang SM et al. PAX6 gene associated with high myopia: A meta-analysis. Optometry Vision Science Official Public American Academy of Optometry. 2014;**91**:419-429

[49] Saw S-M, Matsumura S, Hoang QV. Prevention and management of myopia and myopic pathology. Investigative Ophthalmology & Visual Science. 2019;**60**:488-499

[50] He M et al. Effect of time spent outdoors at school on the development of myopia among children in China: A Randomized Clinical Trial. JAMA. 2015;**314**:1142-1148

[51] Popov I et al. Effect of blue light filtering intraocular lenses on visual perception. Medicina (Mex.). 2021;**57**(559)

[52] Huang J et al. Efficacy comparison of 16 interventions for myopia control in children: A network meta-analysis. Ophthalmology. 2016;**123**:697-708

[53] Chia A et al. Atropine for the treatment of childhood myopia: Changes after stopping atropine 0.01%, 0.1% and 0.5%. American Journal of Ophthalmology. 2014;**157**:451-457

[54] Chia A, Lu Q-S, Tan D. Five-year clinical trial on atropine for the treatment of Myopia 2: Myopia control with atropine 0.01% eyedrops. Ophthalmology. 2016;**123**:391-399

[55] Lam CSY, Tang WC, Tse DY-Y, Tang YY, To, C. H. Defocus Incorporated Soft Contact (DISC) lens slows myopia progression in Hong Kong Chinese schoolchildren: A 2-year randomised clinical trial. The British Journal of Ophthalmology. 2014;**98**:40-45

[56] Chamberlain P et al. A 3-year randomized clinical trial of misight lenses for myopia control. Optometry and Vision Science Official Publication American Academy of Optometry. 2019;**96**:556-567

[57] Correction of Myopia Evaluation Trial 2 Study Group for the Pediatric Eye Disease Investigator Group. Progressive-addition lenses versus single-vision lenses for slowing progression of myopia in children with high accommodative lag and near esophoria. Investigative Ophthalmology and Visual Science. 2011;**52**:2749-2757

[58] Cheng D, Woo GC, Drobe B, Schmid KL. Effect of bifocal and prismatic bifocal spectacles on myopia progression in children: Three-year results of a randomized clinical trial. JAMA Ophthalmology. 2014;**132**:258-264

Section 3

Corneal Refractive Surgery

Chapter 3

Modern Refractive Lenticular Femtosecond Laser Corneal Surgery for Correction of Myopia and Myopic Astigmatism

Maja Bohač, Mateja Jagić, Doria Gabrić, Lucija Zerjav, Smiljka Popović Suić and Iva Dekaris

Abstract

Small-incision lenticule extraction (SMILE) is becoming the procedure of choice in treating myopia and myopic astigmatism. With great comparability in terms of visual outcome with the femtosecond laser-assisted in situ keratomileusis (FsLASIK) procedure, the method is characterized by better patient satisfaction and less postoperative dry eye induction. Moreover, it has the advantages of better eye surface stability and biomechanical strength compared to FS-LASIK. The method is now globally accepted among refractive surgeons. Patients suitable for the procedure must meet criteria for keratorefractive procedures generally. Our current clinical experience suggests that the lenticule extraction procedure delivers promising refractive results in terms of predictability, efficacy, and safety.

Keywords: lenticule extraction, SMILE, LASIK, femtosecond laser, myopia, refractive surgery

1. Introduction

LASIK is the most commonly used corneal refractive surgical procedure to treat ametropia worldwide [1, 2]. Compared to earlier microkeratome variant, femtosecond laser-assisted laser in situ keratomileusis (FsLASIK) provides precise flap creation achieving better morphological stability. Even so, flap related complications, induction of higher-order aberrations, as well as biomechanical corneal instability are still present [3–5]. When ablating stroma between 10 and 30% of depth, LASIK is estimated to reduce the tensile strength of the stroma by about 35% [6–8].

In recent years, the lenticle extraction method has gradually become popular as a potential alternative for traditional LASIK and PRK procedures. The femtosecond laser-assisted corneal procedure known as small-incision lenticule extraction (SMILE) was first described by Sekundo et al. in 2008 [9] and after larger series followed, the procedure became clinically available in 2011. Using an ultrashort pulse laser system, procedure delineates contour of tissue volume that needs to be excised in order to accomplish refractive correction. It is a flapless procedure where two precise intrastromal planar sections are created by femtosecond laser forming the lenticule that is manually extracted through a superiorly (nasal/temporal) placed small 2–5 mm length incision after careful dissection from the pocket. When removing intrastromal lenticule, corneal shape is altered without Bowman's membrane disruption, therefore procedure offers biomechanical stability of the cornea, especially in treatment of higher levels of myopia and astigmatism [6, 9]. Since there is no flap creation, lenticule extraction procedure rules out formerly known risks in LASIK procedures, such as flap creation complication and dislocation [6–8, 10–12].

2. Small-incision lenticule extraction

Recently, two emerging alternatives have been introduced in the market: CLEAR using Z8 by Ziemer, Switzerland [13–15] and SmartSight using ATOS by SCHWIND eye-tech-solutions, Germany [16, 17].

CLEAR (Corneal Lenticule Extraction for Advanced Refractive correction) treatment is an additional treatment program from FEMTO LDV Z8, which is a multipurpose laser (cataract surgery, corneal transplantation, flap creation for LASIK, tunnel/pocket creation for inlays, arcuate incision). In the technical aspect, it works under pulse energies below 100 nJ with a repetition rate above 20 MHz and a spiral raster laser pattern [15]. Besides eye-tracking guided centration, the laser system has intraoperative OCT, which is predominantly used for cases of corneal transplantation, tunnel creation for inlays, and cataract surgery. The ability to create two side-cuts potentially reduces the learning curve for less experienced surgeons since tunnels guide directly to the anticipated plane of the lenticule (anterior or posterior) [13, 14].

SmartSight treatment profile by SCHWIND ATOS, without using side cuts, does not have a minimal thickness (as in SMILE) and includes lenticule tapering toward the periphery, a refractive progressive transition zone, to achieve minimal refractive regression by reducing epithelial remodelling [17]. The laser works in the plasma-mediated ablation regime, slightly above the threshold for laser-induced optical breakdown, and below the photodisruption regime. It works under pulse energy below 100 nJ, with spot spacing >4 μm and track spacing ~3 μm, with a repetition rate up to 4 MHz, and an asymmetric scanning pattern. The laser system has cyclotorsion control, where it incorporates a video-based eye registration from the diagnostic image along with an eye-tracker guided centration to improve the predictability of the astigmatic corrections (**Figure 1**).

When forming and extracting lenticule in SMILE procedure from anterior half of the stroma, the tensile corneal strength is reduced by 55% while this effect is less profound in the case of lenticule formed in deeper stromal layers [7]. Therefore, extent of changes in biomechanical corneal properties is depending on the lenticule volume and location (depth) in the cornea [7, 8, 18].

The differences between SMILE and FsLASIK are potential sources that could influence the final refractive and overall optical performance of the eye after surgery by inducing unwanted astigmatism. Moreover, there has been an increasing awareness and understanding of the change in higher-order optical aberrations following corneal refractive surgery over the last two decades. It is widely accepted

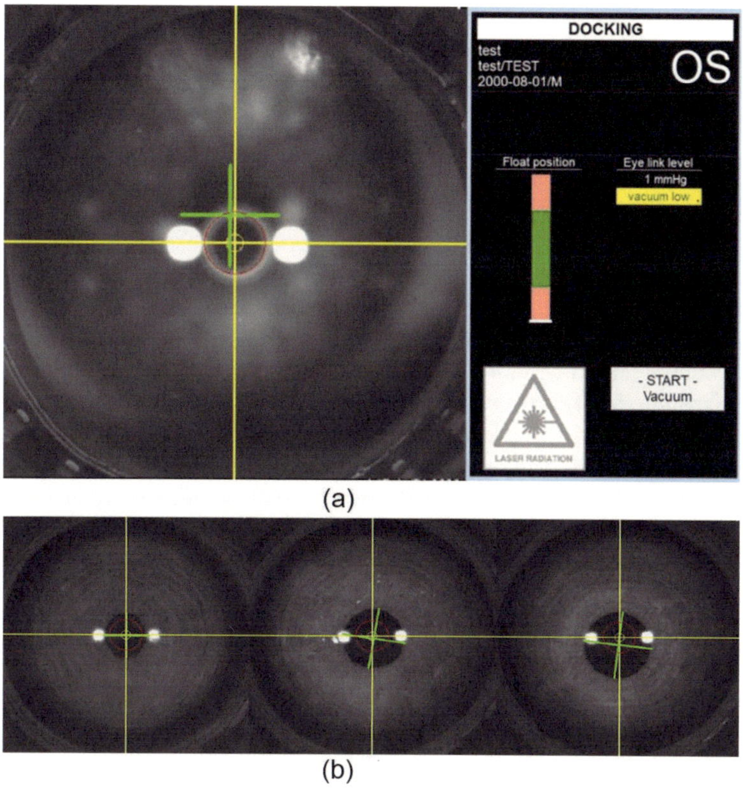

Figure 1.
Video-based eye registration (cyclotorsion control) from the diagnostic image along with an eye-tracker guided centration inside the Schwind ATOS.

that higher-order aberrations should be either maintained after surgery at preoperative levels or modified to improve the overall optical and visual performances of the eye [19–22].

2.1 Indications

Indications for lenticule extraction adhere to the guidelines for all corneal refractive surgical procedures [23].

Prior to the decision if the patient meets the criteria for refractive surgery complete ophthalmologic examination is needed. The examination includes uncorrected distance visual acuity, corrected distance visual acuity, manifest and cycloplegic refraction, corneal tomography, corneal and ocular aberrometry, tonometry, slit lamp, and dilated funduscopic examination.

Patients with stable refraction, myopia up to −10.00 D, and astigmatism up to 5 D or SE up to 12.50 D with sufficient corneal thickness and normal tomography are considered eligible candidates. As the most common contraindications would be considered: abnormal corneal topography, signs of progressive preoperative corneal thickness <480 μm or calculated residual stromal bed thickness <275 μm, scotopic pupil wider than 7.5 mm, dry eye, inflammation of ocular adnexa and periocular area, active autoimmune disease or connective tissue diseases.

2.2 Surgical procedure

The surgery is performed under topical anesthesia. After standardized cleaning with 2.5% povidone-iodine and sterile draping, an eyelid speculum is used to keep the eye open. After positioning patient on the surgical bed, and connecting the surgical cone (disposable interface) to suction ports, the patient is instructed to fixate the light target when the eye is aligned with the cone. When centration coincides with the visual axis and there is visible matching of corneal vertex (from corneal tomography), suction can be applied, followed by treatment initialization and laser ablation immediately after complete suction is achieved. Caps can be 100–150 μm thick and incisions are usually positioned superotemporal with width between 2.5 and 3.2 mm. The optical zone selected depends on the scotopic pupil size and attempted correction. Automatic suction release occurs upon completion of lenticule formation. After identifying both anterior and posterior lenticular surface with thin blunt spatula, separation of the lenticule and extraction through the side cut is performed. In order to detect any residual material or tears, lenticule tissue is thoroughly inspected.

2.3 Clinical results

In two separated studies we were evaluating outcomes, safety, efficacy, and predictability of small-incision lenticule extraction procedures performed at different laser systems. For treating myopia and myopic astigmatism. In first study, ReLEx SMILE procedure was performed on VisuMax from Zeiss, with comparing refractive and visual outcomes with FsLASIK procedure performed on VisuMax for flap creation and Schwind Sirius 750s for excimer ablation at one-year period. The second study was conducted on Atos for Schwind eye-tech-solutions, performing SmartSight lenticule extraction procedure. During a three-month follow up refractive, wavefront, and topographic outcomes were evaluated. The results of both studies are presented below.

2.3.1 Smile vs FS LASIK

2.3.1.1 Astigmatism

There was a significant difference in the magnitude of astigmatism between the SMILE and the FsLASIK groups one year after the surgery [24]. Postoperatively, the amount of any astigmatism revealed by subjective refraction results from a combination of the treated astigmatism coupled with the effects of postoperative healing. In the SMILE group, we encountered more residual manifest astigmatism compared with the FsLASIK group. Vector analysis of astigmatism did not show any difference between the two groups prior to surgery. Both mean J_0 and J_{45} values were slightly lower in the FsLASIK group in comparison with the SMILE group indicating that astigmatism is less prevalent after FsLASIK (**Figures 2–5**). This indication is further supported by the slightly higher surgically induced astigmatism values following SMILE compared with FsLASIK. Both techniques of vector analysis show that individual differences between the vector value pre- and postoperative were strongly correlated with the preoperative vector values. This is encouraging indicating that for individual cases the postoperative astigmatic vector values can be predicted with precision using the preoperative astigmatic value in both SMILE and FsLASIK. The Thibos' method of vector analysis [25], clearly points out that within the SMILE

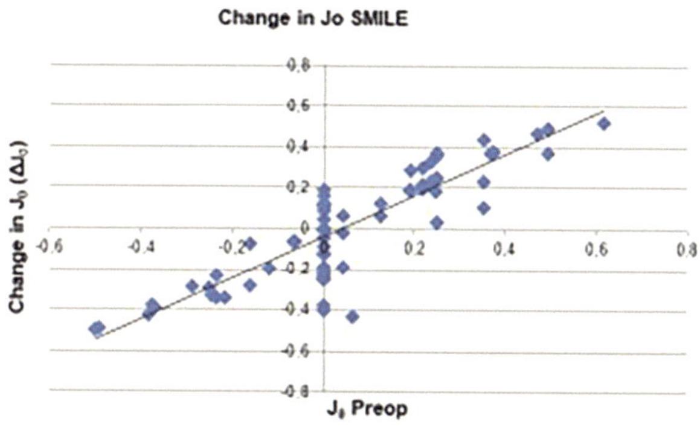

Figure 2.
Change in J_0 vector value in each case treated with SMILE procedure. Significant association between the change in J_0 (ΔJ_0) and preop J_0 value presented as linear regression. The least squares line: $\Delta J_0 = 1.015 J_0 + 0.040$ ($R = .861$, $N = 89$, $P < .001$).

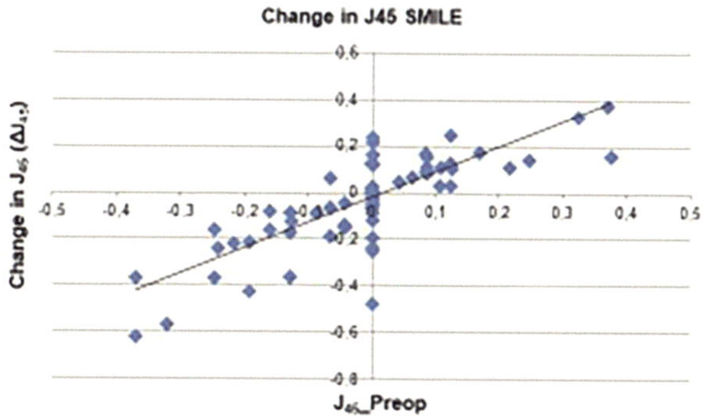

Figure 3.
Change in J_{45} vector value in each case treated with SMILE procedure. Significant association between the change in J_{45} (ΔJ_{45}) and preop J_{45} value is presented as linear regression. The least squares line: $\Delta J_{45} = 1.082 J_{45} + 0.019$ ($R = .792$, $N = 89$, $P < .001$).

group the correlation between ΔJ_{45} and preoperative J_{45} (0.792) tended to be lower in comparison with the counterpart in the FsLASIK group (0.924). This suggests that the precision of controlling a change in astigmatism with FsLASIK is superior compared with SMILE.

Turning to the mean target and surgically induced astigmatism values, in the FsLASIK group the target and surgically induced astigmatism values were nearly identical. This can only occur when the residual astigmatism is almost totally nullified. In the SMILE group, the mean surgically induced astigmatism was significantly higher than the target induced astigmatism (−0.57 D and −0.41 D respectively). This indicates that the SMILE procedure tends to overcorrect and even induce astigmatism. The centration is different for both SMILE and FsLASIK procedures, wherein SMILE, procedure is centred on the visual axis and FsLASIK is centred on the corneal vertex. In the event that the intersection of the corneal surface and the visual axis does not coincide with corneal apex, a smaller amount of unwanted astigmatism may be predicted [26]. Given the procedure centration on corneal vertex, this should more likely occur after FsLASIK. Other factors must be responsible for the increased astigmatism after SMILE.

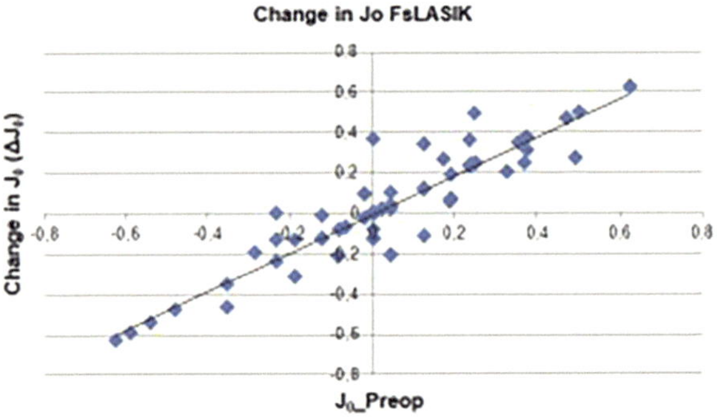

Figure 4.
Change in J_0 vector value in each case treated with FsLASIK procedure. Significant association between the change in J_0 (ΔJ_0) and preop J_0 value is presented as linear regression. The least squares line: $\Delta J_0 = 0.952J_0 - 0.005$ ($R = .921$, $N = 92$, $P < .001$).

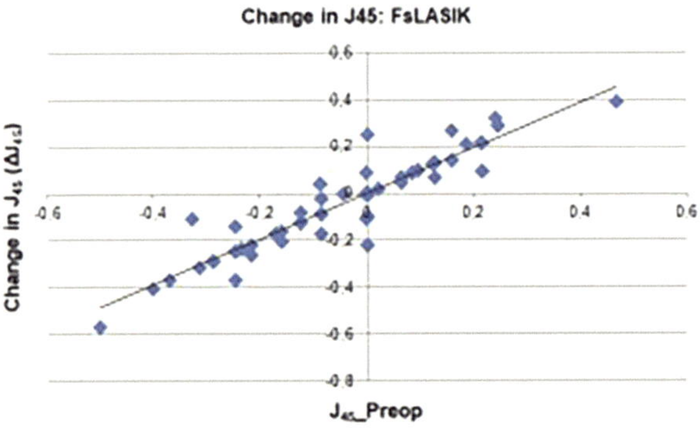

Figure 5.
Change in J_{45} vector value in each case treated with FsLASIK procedure. Significant association between the change in J_{45} (ΔJ_{45}) and preop J_{45} value. Is presented as linear regression. The least squares line: $\Delta J_{45} = 0.962J_{45} - 0.002$ ($R = .923$, $N = 92$, $P < .001$).

In **Figures 6** and 7 vector diagrams demonstrate the unwanted induced astigmatism that occurred in some cases, where surgically induced astigmatism values appear more dispersed from the central point in the SMILE group compared with the FsLASIK group. Of a total of 89 eyes treated with SMILE procedure, at one-year postop we found three cases where astigmatism increased by 0.75 D and 10 cases where astigmatism increased by 0.50 D. The results of astigmatic corrections after SMILE differ among authors. Some authors reported no significant differences in postoperative astigmatism between SMILE and FsLASIK, and no significant increases in astigmatism [27, 28]. On the other hand, others reported more favourable outcomes after FsLASIK [29]. In addition, Kunert et al. [30] and Qian et al. [31] reported up to 1.00 D overcorrection of astigmatism and an overall undercorrection of high astigmatism after the SMILE procedure. None of the available reports mentions or discusses cases where astigmatism becomes manifest during the postop period. Unexpected postoperative astigmatism following a SMILE procedure could, to some extent, be explained by insufficient intraoperative centration, decentration of refractive lenticule ablation profile relative to the visual axis, dislodged fragments from the lenticule (although we did not encounter any), and the impact of any epithelial hyperplasia

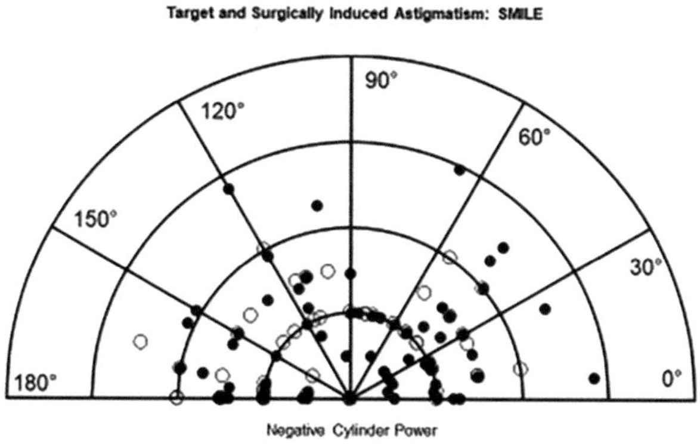

Figure 6.
Polar diagram showing target and surgically induced astigmatic values for the SMILE group. The targeted surgically induced astigmatism data points are shown as empty circles and filled dots respectively, with semicircles from −2 DC to 0 (central point) in 0.5DC steps and from 0°to 90°and 180° (right to left) in 30° steps.

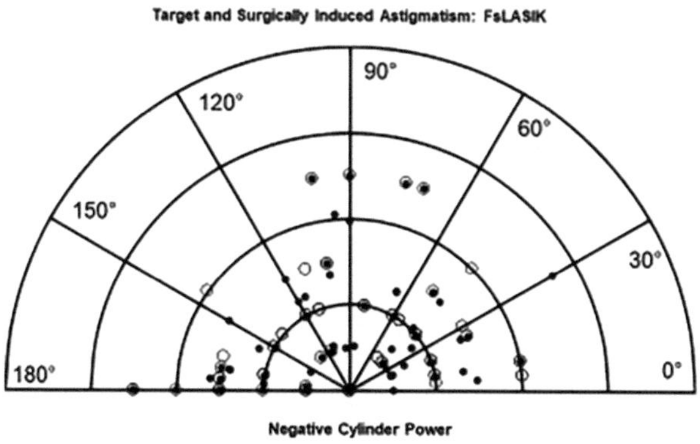

Figure 7.
Polar diagram showing target and surgically induced astigmatic values for the FsLASIK group. The target and surgically induced astigmatism data points are shown as empty circles and filled dots respectively, with semicircles from −2 DC to 0 (central point) in 0.5DC steps and from 0°to 90°and 180° (right to left) in 30° steps.

during the postoperative period. The lower incidence of astigmatism in the FsLASIK group may be linked to the advanced eye-tracking devices designed to compensate for any cyclotorsional effect and eye movements during the excimer laser ablation [32]. For the SMILE procedure centration was achieved manually after instructing the patient to fixate a blinking green light and locking the laser procedure about the visual axis using suction ports [6]. Slight tilting of the lenticule, in association with any decentration, would further contribute to any unexpected postop astigmatism.

2.3.1.2 Higher order aberrations (HOAs)

At one-year postop, significant differences between the two groups were found for all higher-order aberrations (HOAs). Coma, trefoil, and spherical aberration (SA) tended to be lower in the FsLASIK group compared with SMILE. In the SMILE group, a significant increase in postoperative SA was revealed while there were no differences for coma or trefoil. For the FsLASIK group, significant changes in coma and trefoil were observed but not for SA. The changes in the mean values of some HOAs were statistically significant, but their clinical relevance is open to question. **Figures 8–13** show there are highly significant correlations between changes in coma, trefoil, and SA in individual cases when compared with preoperative values. The results of these linear regressions can be used to predict the likely change in an HOA we can expect to encounter after surgical intervention on an individual case-by-case basis. For example, **Figures 8** and **9** show preoperative values for coma below 0.15 μm are not expected to change greatly after either SMILE or FsLASIK. The magnitude of coma is predicted to fall by approximately 0.14 μm after either procedure when the preop value is in the region of 0.30 μm. Turning to **Figures 12** and **13**, when the preoperative SA is of the order +0.10 μm the postoperative value should reduce by nearly 50% after either SMILE or FsLASIK. However, if the preoperative was −0.10 μm the predicted postoperative value after SMILE is +0.010 μm and +0.002 μm after FsLASIK. Thus, when refractive surgery is the desired option, it would be advisable to treat highly aberrated eyes with FsLASIK.

Our results conflict with other published reports. Wu et al. [33] reported the magnitude of all higher-order aberrations increased after either SMILE or FsLASIK. However, after surgery, the average values for SA and horizontal coma were lower in the SMILE group compared with the FsLASIK group. Lin et al. [34] also reported increases in all ocular higher-order aberrations after both SMILE and FsLASIK but, with significantly lower values of SA and coma after the SMILE procedure. Others report that contrast sensitivity improved after SMILE implying more favorable high order aberration profiles [6, 28]. Our experience does not support previous reports because we found SA increased after SMILE with coma and trefoil reduction after the FsLASIK. The differences between some reports may be due to several factors such as geographical factors. For example, the work of Wu et al. [33] Lin et al. [34], and Liu et al. [35] were based in Southeast Asia, and the work by Ganesh et al. [36] was based in India. Our results were obtained predominantly from Caucasian eyes. The differences in the outcomes between studies can result from a variety of reasons including genetic factors. However, results based on studies in other territories are concordant with the findings from Asia [6, 27, 37].

2.3.1.3 Conclusion

In conclusion, our experience with both procedures yields satisfactory visual acuity results. However, FsLASIK offers a marginally improved outcome as indicated by the residual high order aberrations and astigmatism.

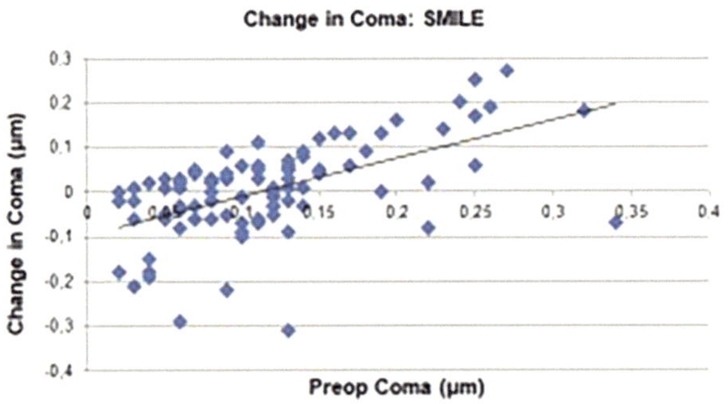

Figure 8.
Change in coma value in each case treated with SMILE procedure. Significant association between the change in coma (y) and preop coma (x) value presented as linear regression. The least squares line: y = 0.847x − 0.094 (R = .562, N = 89, P < .001).

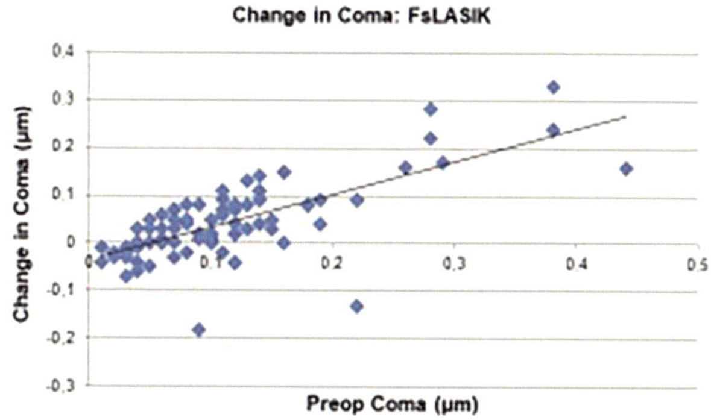

Figure 9.
Change in coma value in each case treated with FsLASIK procedure. Significant association between the change in coma (y) and preop coma (x) value presented as linear regression. The least squares line: y = 0.688x − 0.034 (R = .743, N =92, P < .001).

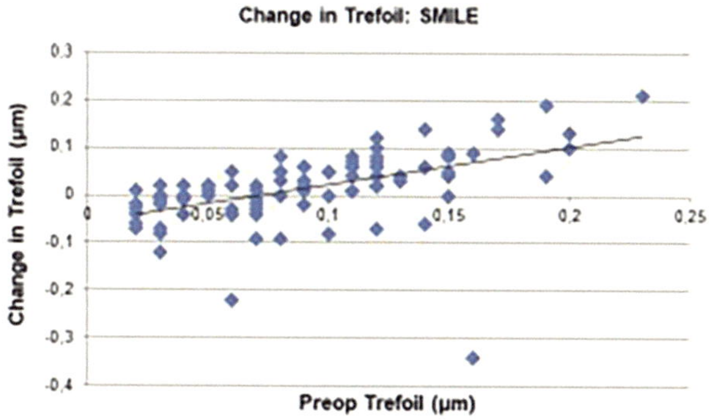

Figure 10.
Change in trefoil value in each case treated with SMILE procedure. Significant association between the change in trefoil (y) and preop trefoil (x) value presented as linear regression. The least squares line: y = 0.793x − 0.057 (r = .515, N = 89, P < .001).

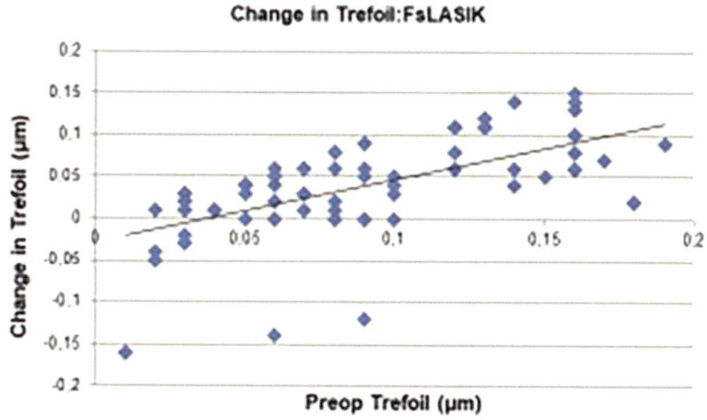

Figure 11.
Change in trefoil value in each case treated with FsLASIK procedure. Significant association between the change in trefoil (y) and preop trefoil (x) value presented as linear regression. The least squares line: y = 0.741x − 0.027 (R = .618, N = 92, P < .001).

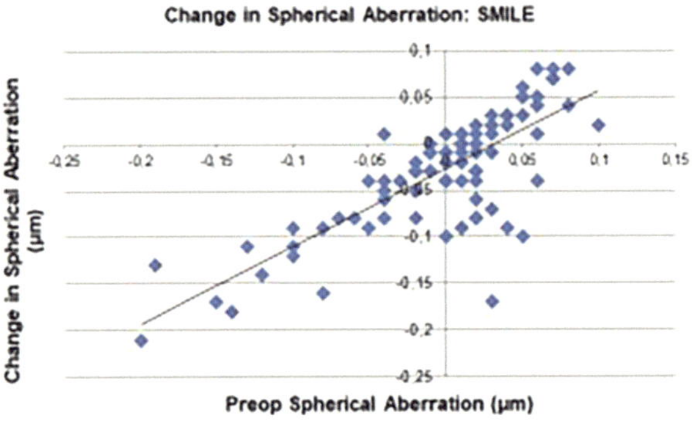

Figure 12.
Change in spherical aberration (SA) value in each case treated with SMILE procedure. Significant association between the change in SA (y) and preop SA (x) value presented as linear regression. The least squares line: $y = 0.832x - 0.027$ ($R = .779$, $N = 89$, $P < .001$).

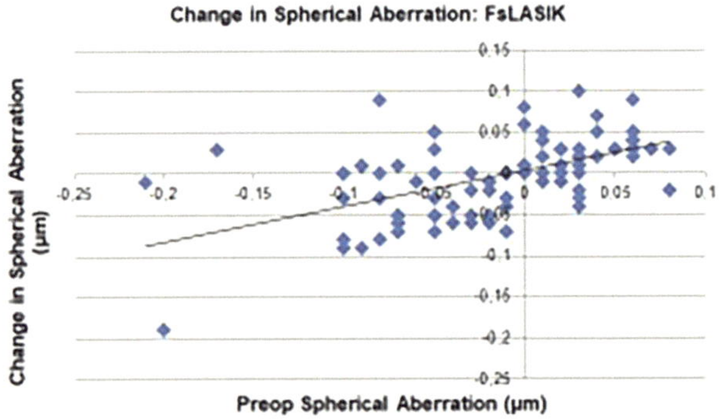

Figure 13.
Change in spherical aberration (SA) value in each case treated with FsLASIK procedure. Significant association between the change in SA (y) and preop SA (x) value presented as linear regression. The least squares line: $y = 0.428x + 0.004$ ($R = .545$, $N = 92$, $P < .001$).

2.3.2 SmartSight lenticule extraction on SCHWIND ATOS

2.3.2.1 Efficacy and safety

The short-term changes at three-month follow-up of the efficacy and safety of lenticule extraction treatments using the SmartSight profile were analyzed.

The main difference and advantage of SCHWIND ATOS and SmartSight at this time of development is the low energy delivered to the cornea since the laser works slightly above the threshold for the laser-induced optical breakdown with energies between 80 and 100 nJ. In addition, the laser also possesses features such as cyclotorsion control and eye-tracker guided centration. Lack of the abovementioned technologies was one of the main drawbacks for the surgeons in transition from excimer laser-based procedures to lenticular extraction and was often emphasized as the main shortcoming in the treatment of a higher amount of astigmatism.

The analysis revealed promising results after the treatment. The unaided vision was expected to improve overall. Most of the outcome measures showed significant improvement compared to the preoperative status. The improvement in visual acuities was significant (**Figures 14–16**).

2.3.2.2 Refractive outcome and keratometry

An excellent refractive outcome was observed in terms of manifest refraction, but this was only partly confirmed by the objective refraction and the topographical changes. This suggests that manifest refraction may be more forgiving in terms of exactly determining the accuracy of the treatments, but at the same time, UDVA is the main driver for patient satisfaction. CDVA loss of two lines occurred only in a single eye (**Figure 17**).

At three months after the surgery, for the change in wavefront refraction or corneal keratometry 68% of eyes were within 0.5D from target (**Figures 18** and **19**), with 63% and 58% of eyes within 0.5D from target astigmatism for wavefront refraction and corneal keratometry, respectively (**Figures 20** and **21**). The angle of error was within 25° from the attempted astigmatism axis in 60% and 42% of the eyes for wavefront refraction and corneal keratometry, respectively (**Figure 22**).

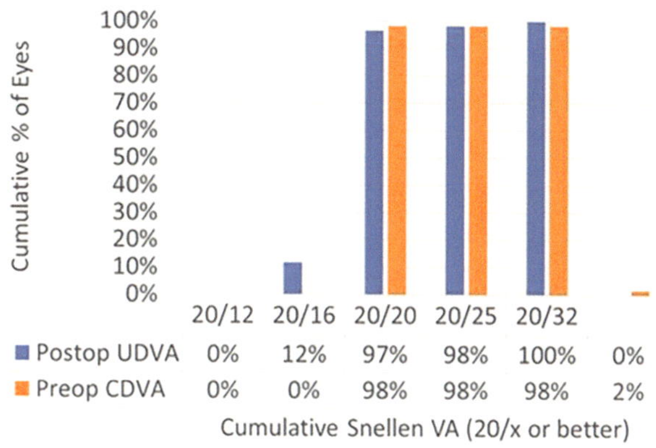

Figure 14.
Standard graphs for reporting outcomes in laser vision correction: Cumulative Snellen Visual acuity.

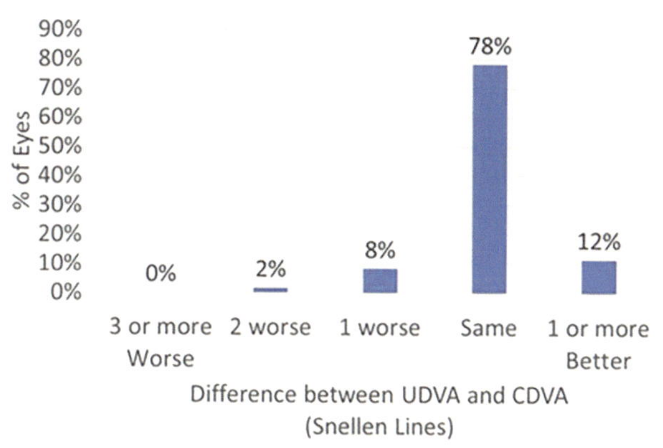

Figure 15.
Difference between UDVA and CDVA.

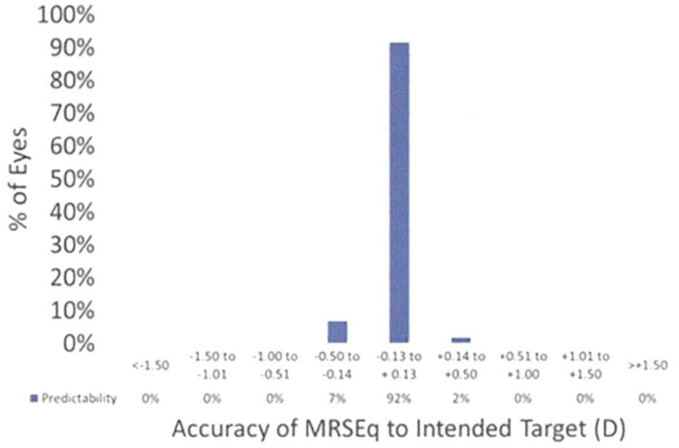

Figure 16.
Accuracy of MRSEq to intended target (D).

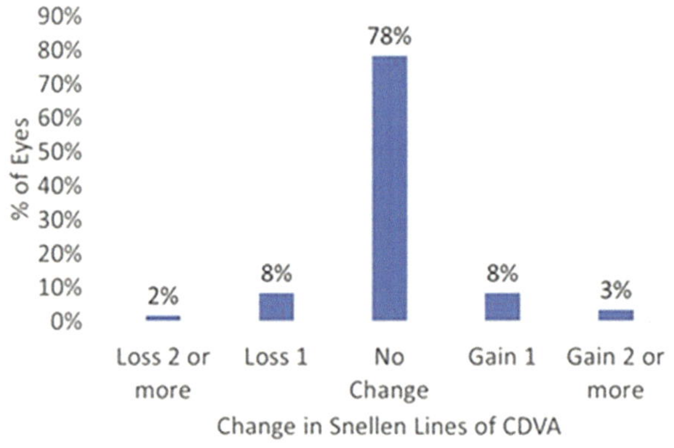

Figure 17.
Change in Snellen lines of CDVA.

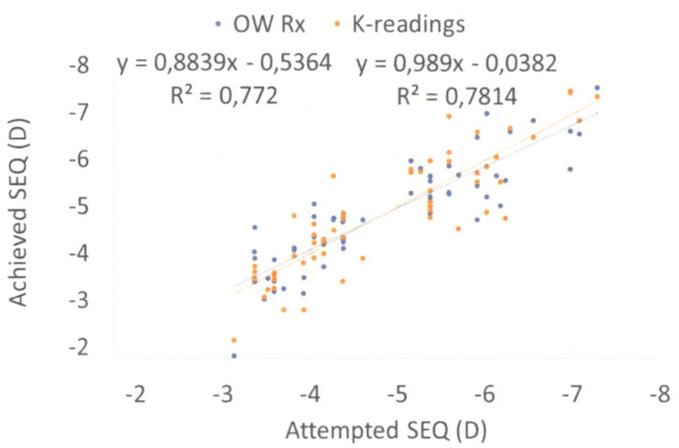

Figure 18.
Wavefront refraction vs. attempted SEQ (D).

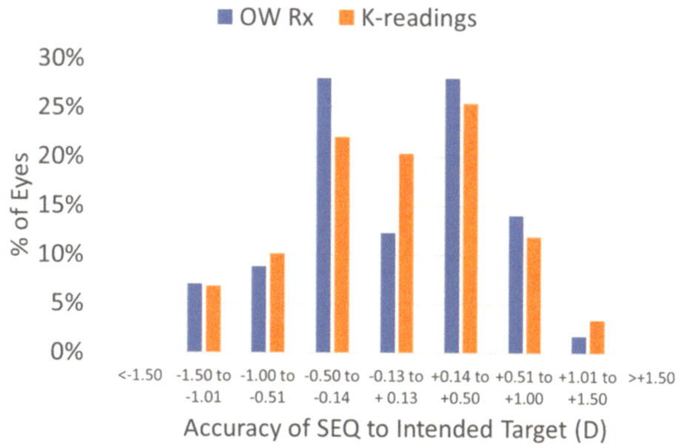

Figure 19.
Accuracy of SEQ to intended target (D).

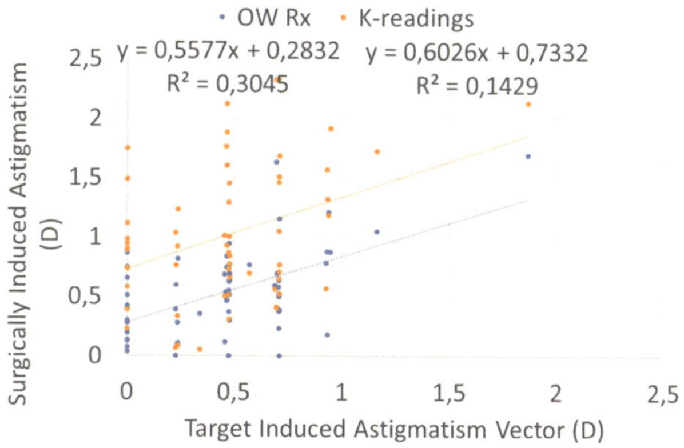

Figure 20.
Scattergram of achieved change in wavefront refraction vs attempted correction of the astigmatism.

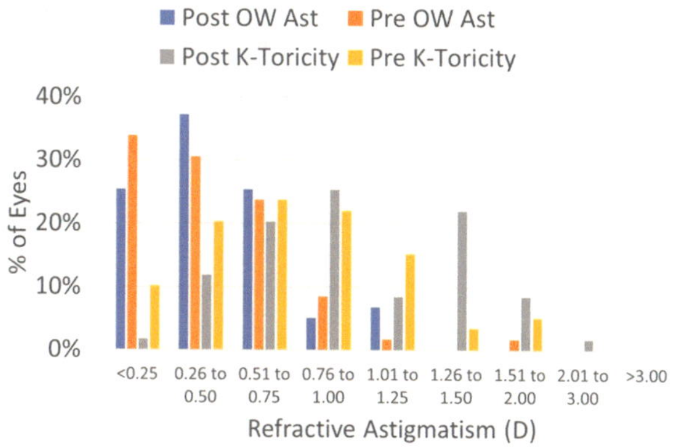

Figure 21.
Percentage of eyes within intended target of postoperative astigmatism.

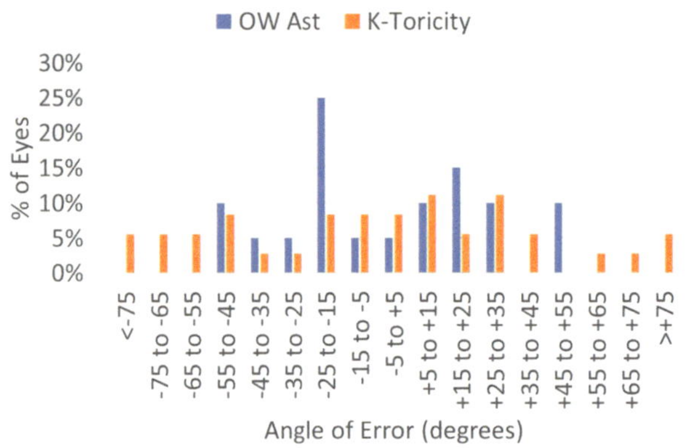

Figure 22.
Angle of error from attempted astigmatism axis.

Previous publications, like recent studies by Sideroudi et al. [38] and Ganesh et al. [39], suggest that undercorrection in SMILE can be associated with forward shifting of posterior corneal surface that leads to posterior curvature steepening. Opposite to our findings, some works report lower changes observed in keratometries than in refraction. This could be due to using simpler models and not considering difference in refractive indices (used for keratometry) and actual refractive corneal index, the effect of central tissue removal on refraction, or effect of the vertex distance on planned refraction (spectacle plane to corneal plane). Taking this into consideration, The SmartSight profile involves tapering the lenticule toward the edge to achieve smoothing of the transition zone from treated to the untreated cornea in an attempt to reduce the biomechanical changes and epithelial remodelling on the edge of the treatment. It is determined as refractive progressive transition zone, similar to the one used in the SCHWIND AMARIS ablation profiles, ranging from 0.2 mm to 0.8 mm, determined by corneal curvature gradient and also induced by correction.

In this study at three months, the scattergram of achieved change in wavefront refraction vs. achieved change in keratometry readings of the SEQ showed a very good correlation (**Figure 23**), with 75% eyes within 0.75D (**Figure 24**).

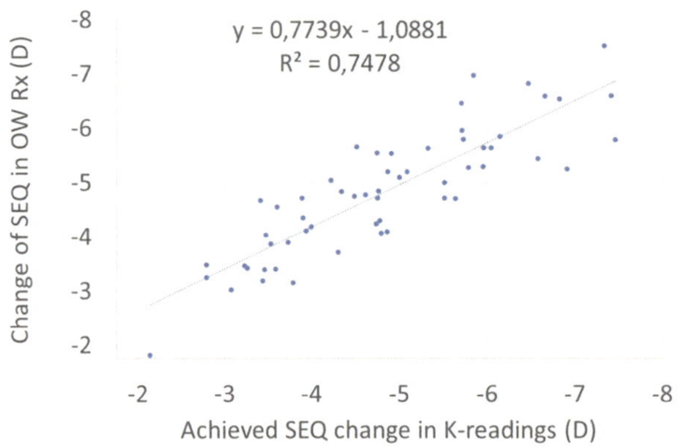

Figure 23.
Scattergram of achieved change in wavefront refraction vs achieved change in keratometry readings of the SEQ.

2.3.2.3 Corneal and ocular wavefront (aberrations)

Corneal aberrations slightly increased after the treatment, but the change of ocular aberrations was very minor and non-significant (**Figures 25** and **26**). This may confirm the relatively neutral behaviour in terms of aberrations reported from other refractive lenticule extraction techniques, as well as be indicative of adequate centration. SA was less positive when measured with ocular aberrations than for corneal aberrations. Postoperative corneal SA increased more than ocular SA, remaining stable at three months follow-up. The RMS higher-order aberrations increased, both for corneal and ocular aberrations, with corneal aberrations showing systematically higher inductions HOA than the ocular counterparts (**Figure 27**). Corneal topography and aberrometry revealed an induction of positive SA associated with an increase in the RMS higher-order aberrations.

2.3.2.4 Conclusion

A limitation of this work is that only 50 eyes of 31 consecutive patients completed the three-months follow-up and were included for analyses. Another limitation is the retrospective nature of the study. Several confounding factors may be argued in our review, we have considered both eyes of the patients.

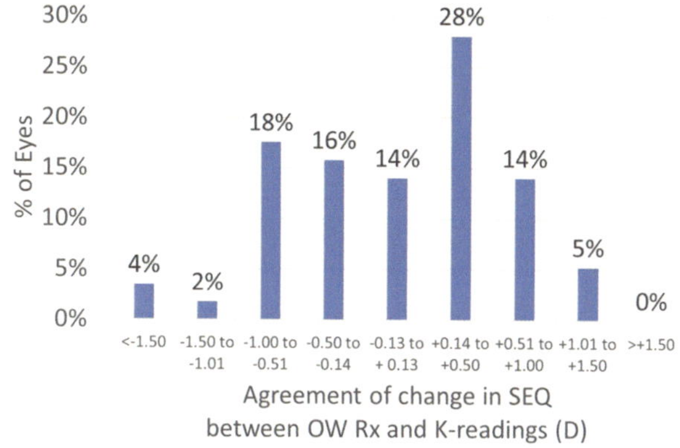

Figure 24.
Agreement of change in SEQ between wavefront refraction and keratometry readings.

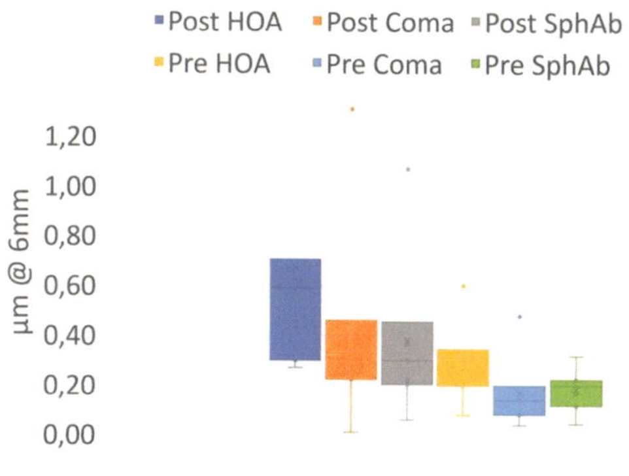

Figure 25.
Preoperative and postoperative corneal wavefront aberrations.

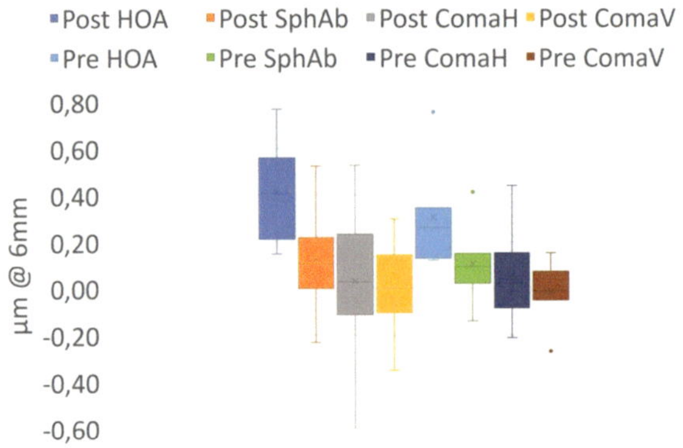

Figure 26.
Preoperative and postoperative ocular wavefront aberrations.

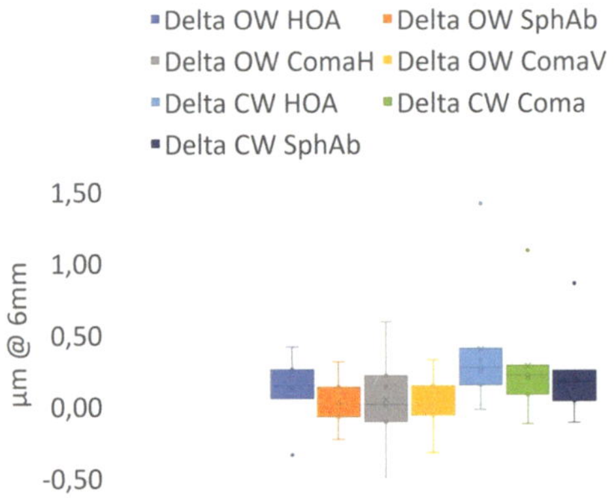

Figure 27.
Change in postoperative HOAs from preoperative baseline.

These clinical results are presented based on a three-month clinical follow-up, which is considered minimal for establishing notable clinical significance in refractive surgery. In literature, however, there are results with shorter follow-ups reported for determining the time-course of visual recovery. Studies with longer follow-ups and a greater number of clinical cases will shed light on the durability of performance and allow for further nomogram refinement to improve outcomes.

3. Conclusions

When achieving excellent clinical visual outcomes in refractive surgery, it is often difficult to demonstrate that novel procedures like lenticule extraction are superior to the standardized LASIK procedure. Up to this point, comparable outcomes in terms of refractive predictability, efficacy, and safety at minimum of three months were found, also theoretical biomechanical advantage of lenticule extraction over Fs. LASIK was described in the literature. Still, a longer learning curve for the surgeons, more frequent suction loss occurrence, prolonged visual recovery, and complicated enhancement treatment have been observed when comparing lenticule extraction to traditional Fs. LASIK. Aforementioned requires further enhancement and refinement of the procedure. Given the increasing clinical use over the last decade, lenticule extraction treatment has continuously been optimized and improved through multiple iterations. Introduction of new laser platforms such as CLEAR and SmartSight, with different energy levels, repetition rates and spot spacing has significantly improved visual outcomes. Precisely, combining high frequency and low energy profile for smooth cutting results in lenticule surface that could provide better clinical performance and optical quality for each laser platform. SmartSight treatment includes even a refractive progressive transition zone tapering the lenticule towards the edge of the transition zone to reduce epithelial remodelling and, therefore refractive regression. Additionally, eye tracking, the centring according to pupil, vertex or defined offset by surgeon, and the video-based cyclotorsion compensation are particularly helpful in astigmatism correction. More studies involving a larger number of patients with longer follow-up will evaluate if new profiles and laser platforms can improve already achieved good visual outcomes after lenticule extraction.

Conflict of interest

The authors declare no conflict of interest.

Appendices and nomenclature

LASIK	laser in situ keratomileusis
SMILE	small-incision lenticule extracton
FsLASIK	femtosecond laser-assisted in situ keratomileusis
PRK	photorefractive keratectomy
CLEAR	corneal lenticule extraction for advanced refractive correction
OCT	optical coherence tomography
D	diopter
DC	diopter cylinder
SE, SEq	spherical equivalent
HOA	higher order aberration
SA	spherical aberration
UDVA	uncorrected distance visual acuity
CDVA	corrected distance visual acuity
RMS	root mean square
OW	ocular wavefront
CW	corneal wavefront
nJ	nano Joule
MHz	mega Hertz
μm	micrometer
J_0	vector of astigmatism power at axis of 90° and 180°, so-called Cartesian or with-the-rule astigmatism
J_{45}	vector of astigmatism power at axis of 45° and 135°, so called oblique astigmatism
ΔJ_{45}	overall change in value of J_{45}
ΔJ_0	overall change in value of J_0
R	value that indicates a linear correlation between variables
P	measure of the probability that an observe difference could have occurred

Author details

Maja Bohač*, Mateja Jagić, Doria Gabrić, Lucija Zerjav, Smiljka Popović Suić and Iva Dekaris
University Eye Hospital Svjetlost, Zagreb, Croatia

*Address all correspondence to: maja.bohac@svjetlost.hr

References

[1] Schmack I, Auffarth G, Epstein D, Holzer M. Refractive surgery trends and practice style changes in Germany over a 3-year period. Journal of Refractive Surgery. 2010;**26**:202-208

[2] Lundström M, Manning S, Barry P, et al. The European Registry of Quality Outcomes for Cataract and Refractive Surgery (EUREQUO): A database study of trends in volumes, surgical techniques and outcomes of refractive surgery. Eye and Vision. 2015;**2**:8. DOI: 10.1186/s40662-015-0019-1

[3] von Jagow B, Kohnen T. Corneal architecture of femtosecond laser and microkeratome flaps imaged by anterior segment optical coherence tomography. Journal of Cataract & Refractive Surgery. 2009;**35**:35-41

[4] Binder PS. Flap dimensions created with IntraLase FS laser. Journal of Cataract & Refractive Surgery. 2004;**30**:26-32

[5] Randleman JB, Woodward M, Lynn MJ, Stulting RD. Risk assessment for ectasia after corneal refractive surgery. Ophthalmology. 2008;**115**:37-50

[6] Reinstein DZ, Archer TJ, Gobbe M. Small incision lenticule extraction (SMILE) history, fundamentals of a new refractive surgery technique and clinical outcomes. Eye and Vision. 2014;**1**:3. DOI: 10.1186/s40662-014-0003-1

[7] Reinstein DZ, Archer TJ, Randleman JB. Mathematical model to compare the relative tensile strength of the Cornea after PRK, LASIK, and small incision lenticule extraction. Journal of Refractive Surgery. 2013;**29**:454-460

[8] Randleman JB, Dawson DG, Grossniklaus HE, et al. Depth-dependent cohesive tensile strength in human donor corneas: Implications for refractive surgery. Journal of Refractive Surgery. 2008;**24**:S85-S89

[9] Sekundo W, Kunert KS, Blum M. Small incision corneal refractive surgery using the small incision lenticule extraction (SMILE) procedure for the correction of myopia and myopic astigmatism: Results of a 6 month prospective study. British Journal of Ophthalmology. 2011;**95**:335-339

[10] Vestergaard AH, Grauslund J, Ivarsen AR, Hjortdal JO. Central corneal sublayer pachymetry and biomechanical properties after refractive femtosecond lenticule extraction. Journal of Refractive Surgery. 2014;**30**:102-108

[11] Agca A, Ozgurhan EB, Demirok A, et al. Comparison of corneal hysteresis and corneal resistance factor after small incision lenticule extraction and femtosecond laser-assisted LASIK: A prospective fellow eye study. Contact Lens & Anterior Eye. 2014;**37**:77-80

[12] Wu D, Wang Y, Zhang L, et al. Corneal biomechanical effects: Small-incision lenticule extraction versus femtosecond laser-assisted laser In Situ keratomileusis. Journal of Cataract & Refractive Surgery. 2014;**40**:963-970

[13] Mehta JS. CLEAR for advanced refractive correction. CRS Today Europe. February 2021

[14] Izquierdo L Jr, Sossa D, Ben-Shaul O, Henriquez MA. Corneal lenticule extraction assisted by a low-energy femtosecond laser. Journal of Cataract & Refractive Surgery. 2020;**46**(9):1217-1221

[15] Fuest M, Mehta JS. Advances in refractive corneal lenticule extraction.

Taiwan Journal of Ophthalmology. 2021;**11**(2):113-121

[16] KR, Arba-Mosquera S. Three-month outcomes of myopic astigmatism correction with small incision guided human Cornea treatment. Journal of Refractive Surgery. 2021;**37**(5):304-311. DOI: 10.3928/1081597X-20210210-02. Epub 2021 May 1

[17] Tsai PS, Blinder P, Migliori BJ, et al. Plasma-mediated ablation: An optical tool for submicrometer surgery on neuronal and vascular systems. Current Opinion in Biotechnology. 2009;**20**(1):90-99

[18] Abahussin M, Hayes S, Knox Cartwright NE, et al. 3D collagen orientation study of the human cornea using X-ray diffraction and femtosecond laser technology. Investigative Ophthalmology & Visual Science. 2009;**50**:5159-5164

[19] Smadja D, Santhiago MR, Mello GR, et al. Corneal high order aberrations after myopic wavefront-optimized ablation. Journal of Refractive Surgery. 2013;**29**:42-48

[20] Schallhorn SC, Farjo AA, Huang D, et al. Wavefront-quided LASIK for the correction of primary myopia and astigmatism: A report by the american academy of ophthalmology. Ophthalmology. 2008;**115**:1249-1261

[21] Benito A, Redondo M, Artal P. Temporal evolution of ocular aberrations following laser in situ keratomileusis. Ophthalmic and Physiological Optics. 2001;**31**:421-428

[22] Kouassi FX, Blaizeau M, Buestel C, et al. Comparison of lasik with femtosecond laser versus Lasik with mechanical microkeratome: Predictability of flap depth, corneal biomechanical effects and optical aberrations. Journal Français d'Ophtalmologie. 2012;**35**:2-8

[23] Sutton G, Lawless M, Hodge C. Laser in situ keratomileusis in 2012: A review. Clinical and Experimental Optometry. 2014;**97**:18-29

[24] Bohac M, Koncarevic M, Dukic A, Biscevic A, Cerovic V, Merlak M, et al. Unwanted astigmatism and high-order aberrations one year after excimer and femtosecond corneal surgery. Optometry and Vision Science. 2018 Nov;**95**(11):1064-1076. DOI: 10.1097/OPX.0000000000001298

[25] Thibos LN, Horner D. Power vector analysis of the optical outcome of refractive surgery. Journal of Cataract & Refractive Surgery. 2001;**27**(1):80-85. DOI: 10.1016/s0886-3350(00)00797-5

[26] Charman WN. Unwanted astigmatism in lenses with a concentric variation in sagittal power. American Journal of Optometry and Physiological Optics. 1982;**59**:997-1001

[27] Zhang J, Wang Y, Chen X. Comparison of moderate- to high-astigmatism corrections using wavefront-guided laser In Situ keratomileusis and small-incision lenticule extraction. Cornea. 2016;**35**:523-530

[28] Reinstein DZ, Carp GI, Archer TJ, Gobbe M. Outcomes of small incision lenticule extraction (SMILE) in low Myopia. Journal of Refractive Surgery. 2014;**30**:812-818

[29] Chan TC, Ng AL, Cheng GP, et al. Vector analysis of astigmatic correction after small-incision lenticule extraction and femtosecond-assisted LASIK for low to moderate myopic astigmatism. British Journal of Ophthalmology. 2016;**100**:553-559

[30] Kunert KS, Russmann C, Blum M, Sluyterman VLG. Vector analysis of myopic astigmatism corrected by femtosecond refractive lenticule extraction. Journal of Cataract & Refractive Surgery. 2013;**39**:759-769

[31] Qian Y, Huang J, Zhou X, Wang Y. Comparison of femtosecond laser small-incision lenticule extraction and laser-assisted subepithelial keratectomy to correct myopic astigmatism. Journal of Cataract & Refractive Surgery. 2015;**41**:2476-2486

[32] Arba Mosquera S, Merayo-Lloves J, de Ortueta D. Clinical effects of pure cyclotorsional errors during refractive surgery. Investigative Ophthalmology & Visual Science. 2008;**49**:4828-4836

[33] Wu W, Wang Y. The correlation analysis between corneal biomechanical properties and the surgically induced higher-order aberrations after small incision lenticule extraction and the femtosecond laser in situ keratomileusis. Journal of Ophthalmology. 2015;**2015**:758196. DOI: 10.1155/2015/758196

[34] Lin F, Xu Y, Yang Y. Comparison of the visual results after SMILE and femtosecond laser-assisted LASIK for myopia. Journal of Refractive Surgery. 2014;**30**:248-254

[35] Liu M, Chen Y, Wang D, et al. Clinical outcomes after SMILE and femtosecond laser-assisted LASIK for myopia and myopic astigmatism: A prospective randomized comparative study. Cornea. 2016;**35**:210-216

[36] Ganesh S, Gupta R. Comparison of visual and refractive outcomes following femtosecond laser assisted LASIK with SMILE in patients with myopia and myopic astigmatism. Journal of Refractive Surgery. 2014;**30**:590-596

[37] Sekundo W, Gertnere J, Bertelmann T, Solomatin I. One-year refractive results, contrast sensitivity, high-order aberrations and complications after myopic small-incision lenticule extraction (ReLEx SMILE). Graefe's Archive for Clinical and Experimental Ophthalmology. 2014;**252**:837-843

[38] Sideroudi H, Lazaridis A, Messerschmidt-Roth A, Labiris G, Kozobolis V, Sekundo W. Corneal irregular astigmatism and curvature changes after small incision lenticule extraction: Three-year follow-up. Cornea. 2018;**37**(7):875-880. DOI: 10.1097/ICO.0000000000001532

[39] Ganesh S, Patel U, Brar S. Posterior corneal curvature changes following refractive small incision lenticule extraction. Clinical Ophthalmology. 2015;**9**:1359-1364. DOI: 10.2147/OPTH.S84354

Chapter 4

When LASIK Goes Wrong or LASIK Complications Dilemmas

Fanka Gilevska, Maja Bohač, Smiljka Popović Suić and Mateja Jagić

Abstract

Laser in situ keratomileusis (LASIK) is one of the most commonly performed refractive surgical procedures. During the last two decades, surgical procedure has evolved, but still, there are several intraoperative and postoperative complications possible. Every young LASIK surgeon spends most of the reading time on LASIK complications. They are not frequent, but you have to know precisely what to do when they happen. This chapter should be a guide, based on literature and experience, on how to deal with intraoperative, early postoperative, and late postoperative complications. This chapter will include managing irregular flaps, buttonholes, and free flaps. The treatment scheme for DLK, epithelial ingrowth, and PISK, and when is the time for flap re-lifting. How frequent should be patients' visits not to miss the complication on time? When is the right time for LASIK reoperation? Post LASIK corneal ectasia and how to perform cross-linking over LASIK. Young surgeons need precise guidelines, not just theoretical treatment options to achieve optimal visual outcomes after LASIK procedure.

Keywords: LASIK, complication, DLK, PISK, epithelial ingrowth, ectasia

1. Introduction

Refractive surgery has made great strides over the last two decades. Technological advances have not only been made at the level of keratorefractive surgery, but also in cataract surgery-the introduction of femtosecond lasers, small incision surgery, and presbyopia-correcting IOLs. LASIK is currently the most commonly performed surgical procedure in refractive surgery. Nowadays, postoperative visual acuity less than 20/20 after refractive surgery has become unacceptable given the growing patients' demands for perfect vision and the fact that the vast majority of patients have 20/20 vision achieved with spectacle or contact lens correction preoperatively. Complications in keratorefractive surgery are extremely rare, and serious side effects occur in less than 0.4% of cases. This chapter will present an overview of all known complications of the LASIK keratorefractive procedure with a recommendation for their management.

2. LASIK complications

2.1 Preoperative complications

2.1.1 Anesthesia

Corneal refractive procedures are performed with topical anesthetic drops (0.5% propacaine, 0.5% tetracaine, and 0.4% oxybuprocaine). Preoperative cleaning of the operative region consists of application of Iodine 5% in the conjunctival fornices for 15 seconds. Both the anesthetic and the iodine may cause epithelial weakening, punctate erosions, or irregular corneal surface. (238) Care about the amount of anesthetic and Iodine used prior to the procedure is essential for the protection of the epithelium. Use of viscous artificial tears during the procedure may interfere with the work of microkeratome and should be avoided [1].

2.1.2 Eyelashes, foil, speculum

Securing the operative surface with transparent adhesive foil over the eyelashes, selection of the appropriate speculum providing enough space for the microkeratome, and choice of the proper microkeratome for the given eye anatomy is very important in creating regular flaps [1].

2.1.3 Conjunctiva

Adequate examination of the whole anterior segment, conjunctiva, limbal region, and fornices is very important precondition for successful surgery. Irregularities in the limbal region, scleral elevations, nevus, and tumor prominence in the region of conjunctiva, limbus, or fornices may cause irregular vacuum suction, pseudosuction, and potential vacuum loss which may result in irregular flap due to improper lamellar incision [1].

2.2 Intraoperative complications

2.2.1 Microkeratome-related complications

Automated microkeratome creates a precise cut on the cornea which represents the flap. It consists of an oscillation blade attached to a head and both work with independent motors (one for the oscillation of the blade, other for the movement forward and backward). The surgeon chooses adequate rings for the different diameters and steepness of the cornea, the thickness of the flap (from 90 to 120 microns), hinge position, and its diameter [2].

2.2.1.1 Incomplete or irregular corneal flap

The incidence of incomplete flap is 0.3–1.2% [3]. Incomplete flap occurs when the microkeratome is stopped before the planned hinge position. Stopping of microkeratome most often occurs due to collisions with eyelids and eyelashes, speculum and/or foil, and due to suction (vacuum) loss during passage. The cause can also be of a mechanical nature-a defect in the dissection head (knife) or in the motor unit of the microkeratome [1, 4, 5]. Irregular flaps often result in lack of enough space for laser ablation, also they carry the risk of profound epithelial ingrowth which can result in corneal scarring in the visual axis or even flap melting.

What shall we do?

Every irregular flap has its own irregular bed underneath. If we leave the flap untouched, smooth healing will result and best corrected visual acuity achieved. If we ablate the bed under the irregular flap, then we create an inadequate match for the flap, and it can result in higher order aberrations and loss of best corrected visual acuity. Flap which has only peripheral irregularities, with a diameter larger than intended ablation area (OZ), procedure can be continued with careful flap reposition, and BSCL is case with epithelial defects.

In a highly irregular and thin flap (usually created by a lamellar cut at or above the Bowman's layer) with an inadequate stromal bed, Bowman membrane remains in the central zone or larger in diameter, the procedure is aborted, and re-treatment is postponed for 3–6 months with setting larger and deeper flap cut then initial [1, 4]. When Bowman membrane remains out of the central zone and is small in diameter, treatment can be continued with additional antimetabolite application (Mytomycine C) for 15 s to prevent the epithelial ingrowth. Surface procedures (PRK) after LASIK can increase the risk for corneal haze formation, but in cases where irregular flap is small, and hinge is positioned in ablation area (OZ), LASIK procedure needs to be aborted and surface ablation is preferred retreatment procedure within 3 months [3].

2.2.1.2 Perforated (buttonhole) flap

The incidence of perforated flap (buttonhole) is 0.1–0.6%, and for too thin flap 0.1–0.4% [6]. Flap perforation occurs when the blade of the microkeratome enters the corneal surface-Bowman membrane and epithelium during the passage, usually in the central part of the flap (**Figure 1**). Too thin flaps occur when the blade of the dissection head does not penetrate deep enough into the cornea but stays close to the surface. Perforated flaps are more common in steep corneas (>46.0 D), and inadequately

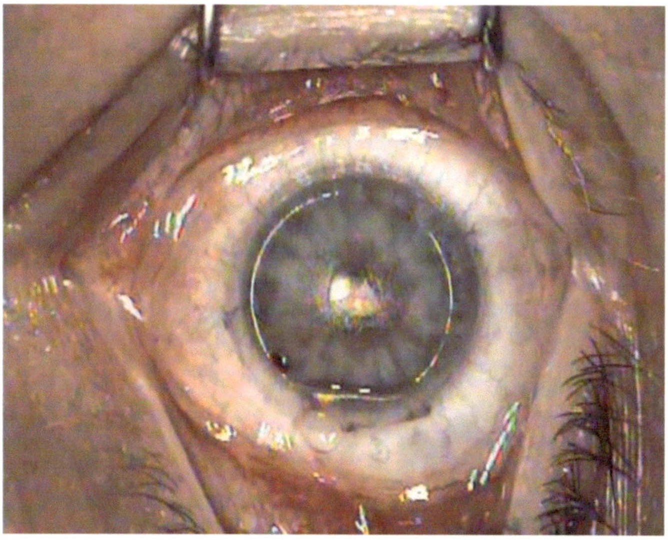

Figure 1.
Intraoperative finding in case of buttonhole flap. Visible central area of Bowmann membrane remains after the flap lift.

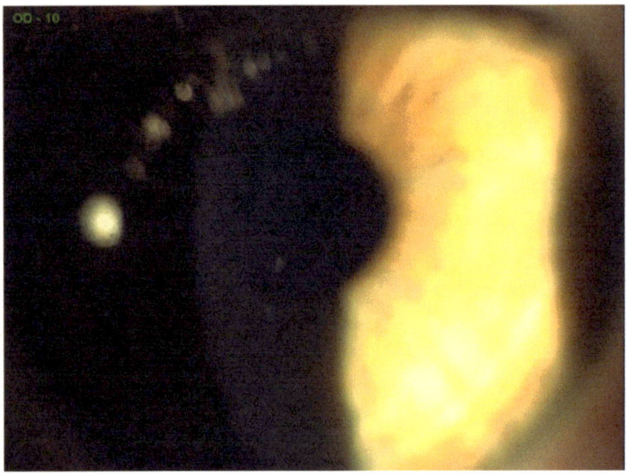

Figure 2.
Post operative finding after reponed flap. In this case procedure was aborted - flap was reposition.

achieved vacuum that causes poor adhesion of the cornea and microkeratome blade, also in flat and small corneas where corneal suction puts cutting plane below the blade [7, 8]. It can also be mechanical in nature due to uneven cutting speed in manual microkeratome, blunt blades, weak blade oscillations, and due to mechanical damage to the blade of the microkeratome dissection head. Perforated flaps are one with the worst visual outcome compared to other intraoperative complications, usually resulting in irregular astigmatism and epithelial ingrowth [1, 7, 8].

What shall we do?

When procedure results in a perforated flap, procedure is aborted, and retreatment is planned after minimum of 3 months, preferably surface ablation (**Figure 2**). In case of LASIK retreatment, a flap with larger diameter and greater thickness should be set [3, 6, 9].

2.2.1.3 Free flap (free cap)

The incidence of free flaps is 0.1–1.0%. The size of the flap depends on the volume of the cornea protruding above the vacuum ring. In the case of protrusion of a small amount of tissue, a free flap is formed. Free flaps are more common in flat corneas with keratometric values <41.0 D, in an insufficient vacuum, when selecting a too small vacuum ring, or in inadequately adjusted microkeratome stoppers [1].

What shall we do?

Adequate cap repositioning on the stromal bed, air dried for at least 3–4 minutes and bandage contact lens placed over for the next few days is crucial for the best visual outcomes. The patient should stay in hospital and be rechecked within 1–2 hours for flap position and its adherence to stromal bed. Dislodging or flap folds that may result from strong eyelid pressure should be treated immediately [1]. In case of excessively edematous flap that tends to dislocate, 10-0 nylon sutures should be used [4]. In case of intraoperative flap loss, procedure is aborted, and after epithelization, refractive error (usually hyperopic shift) can be managed with contact lens or flap reconstruction [10].

2.2.1.4 Corneal perforation

Penetration into the anterior chamber, that is, entry into the anterior chamber with full corneal thickness, may occur during lamellar dissection or even excimer laser photoablation. Perforations can range from simple corneal perforations to perforations with iris and lens damage with or without loss of vitreous. Perforation can occur on extremely thin corneas, in old corneal scars, ulcers, or after previous refractive surgery [1, 11]. Cases with corneal perforation usually have poor visual outcomes due to scar formation and recurrent epithelial ingrowth in perforated plane [12].

What shall we do?

If corneal perforation occurs during flap creation, suction should be immediately stopped. Larger perforation requires surgical repair with suturing under sterile conditions, while small perforations can be managed by flap repositioning and BSCL.

2.2.1.5 Decentered flap

Thin and irregularly decentered flaps can occur during flap formation with both microkeratome or femtosecond laser. The causes are multifactorial and include poor positioning (centering) of the vacuum ring, too low achieved vacuum on the cornea, poor corneal lubrication, poor quality of the blade, pre-existing corneal pathology or microkeratome malfunction [13].

What shall we do?

Since there is likely an unexpected visual outcome after performing centered ablation in a case of decentered flap, it is advised to abort the procedure.

2.2.2 Femtosecond-related complications

The femtosecond laser is a solid-state Nd: Glass laser that works near the infrared spectrum at a wavelength of 1053 nm and produces ultrashort pulses lasting 10–15 s. The laser is based on the principle of nonlinear absorption (corneal tissue is transparent to infrared laser radiation of moderate intensity and without absorption) and the principle of photoionization (laser-induced optical break), which leads to photodisruption. Small tissue volumes are vaporized with the formation of cavitation gas bubbles that gradually disperse into the surrounding tissue and consist of carbon dioxide and water [14–16]. Flap formation is today the most common application of femtosecond lasers, where during clinical practice the superiority of femtosecond lasers over mechanical microkeratomes is slowly indicated in terms of reducing the incidence of intraoperative complications and the ability to personalize switch parameters (diameter, thickness, lateral incision, and hinge) [15, 16].

2.2.2.1 Opaque bubble layer (OBL)

The formation of cavitation bubbles in the lamella between the flap and the stroma, which are directed to the peripheral specially designed pockets, is a standard process of flap formation. In the case of their passage into the deeper stromal layers, or even into the anterior chamber, their confluence occurs, and an opaque layer is formed which interferes with the excimer laser eye tracking system and takes up to several hours to resorb. The penetration of the bubbles into the anterior chamber occurs due to the migration of cavitation bubbles through the 14 piscleral, schlemm canal, and trabecular meshwork into the anterior chamber [17]. Risk factors are thick cornea, small flap diameter, hard docking technique, and low laser frequency or energy [18, 19]. This complication has become very rare since the reduced vacuum pressure on the eye, reduced energy, and increased speed of femtosecond lasers [17, 20–22]. Higher order aberration (HOA) induction, especially trefoil, was reported in cases with OBL [23, 24].

What shall we do?

The presence of OBL suggests flap adhesion so it is advised to perform flap dissection carefully. In case of OBL persistence after flap lift, it will temporarily preclude pupillary tracking for excimer laser ablation. Therefore, waiting for a few minutes and allowing it to disappear is advised. When smaller cavitation bubbles appear in AC, excimer laser treatment can be performed by disabling automatic pupil tracking and proceeding the treatment with manual tracking. Prophylaxis: Setting a larger flap diameter flap and preferring the soft docking technique can reduce the risk of OBL occurrence [18, 19].

2.2.2.2 Vertical gas breakthrough (VBG)

Vertical gas breakthrough (VGB) occurs in the presence of corneal scar or abnormality in the Bowman's layer when the gas dissects vertically towards the stroma or epithelium [25]. When cavitation bubbles penetrate the corneal subepithelial space incomplete flaps or even buttonhole flaps may form while breaching the epithelial layer results in epithelial defect. Bubbles can also penetrate the space between the cornea and the *applanation* lens, preventing laser-treating the cornea. This leads to the formation of tissue bridges and makes it difficult or sometimes impossible to separate the flap from the adjacent stroma. Incidence of VBG is 0.03–0.13% according to the literature [25, 26].

What shall we do?

When the VGB appears, the femtosecond laser treatment should be continued to avoid a partial flap. After assessing the position of the VGB within the flap, further actions are considered: *when* VGB is affecting the visual axis or ahead of the advancing edge of the flap, the flap should not be lifted, and surgery should be aborted [26].

2.2.3 Photoablation-related (excimer laser ablation related) complications

2.2.3.1 Decentered ablation

Centered (over the pupil zone) ablation is crucial for optimal visual outcome, so every deviation in ablation position compromises the visual outcome [4]. Decentration of the ablation zone can occur due to the movement of the laser beam before the excimer laser ablation itself and due to the eye movement during the excimer laser ablation [27].

Decentration is more common in the correction of larger refractive errors (longer excimer laser ablation allows more eye movements), and in patients with poor uncorrected visual acuity who fix the target point even worse due to additional image blur due to corneal dehydration.

During surgery, the decentralized ablation zone may go unnoticed and result in irregular astigmatism and consequent poor visual acuity, dysphotopsia (glare, halo),

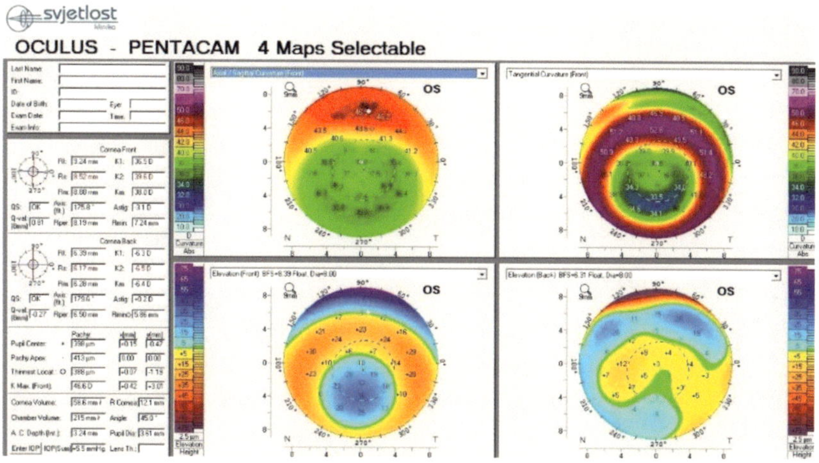

Figure 3.
Decentered ablation after myopic excimer profile.

and monocular diplopia. Usually, it can be presented as asymmetric corneal contour in topography (one side steepening, other side flattening) (**Figure 3**). Decentration can be graded as mild (0–0.5 mm), moderate (0.5–1.0 mm) and severe (>1.0 mm). The magnitude of symptomatic decentration and consequent vision problems varies from patient to patient [1, 27, 28].

What shall we do?

When highly decentered ablation is noticed, with large amount of HOA induction, temporarily miotics can reduce dysphotopsia. After 3 months, customized ablation profiles should be used for retreatment: wavefront- or topo-guided PRK or LASIK procedure [29].

2.2.3.2 Central island

Central islands are diagnosed by corneal topography and are defined as central steep areas of unablated cornea within the treatment zone, defined by their size and keratometric power (>2 mm and > 3D) (**Figure 4**). According to the literature, central island can be considered in every steep corneal zone that affects visual acuity and induces visual disturbances [4, 30]. Central islands are extremely rare in flying spot lasers and can be caused by excimer laser factors (gas dynamics, acoustic corneal shock waves made by laser beams, temporal degradation of laser optics), factors affecting uniform excimer laser delivery like fluid accumulation in the central corneal zone (uneven corneal hydration), and by corneal healing [31]. Central islands cause irregular astigmatism, dysphotopsia (halo, glare, ghost images), loss of best corrected visual acuity, decrease in contrast sensitivity, and monocular diplopia [1, 32].

What shall we do?

It is advised to wait for at least 6 months for stabilization of corneal topography and refractive status since vast majority of central island cases regress spontaneously (up to 80%). If there is a retreatment procedure required, wavefront- or topo-guided ablation profile needs to be planned, since irregular and complex corneal topography [33]. In cases of extremely irregular topography and risk of ending with questionable results of retreatment, rigid-gas permeable lenses can be used for correction.

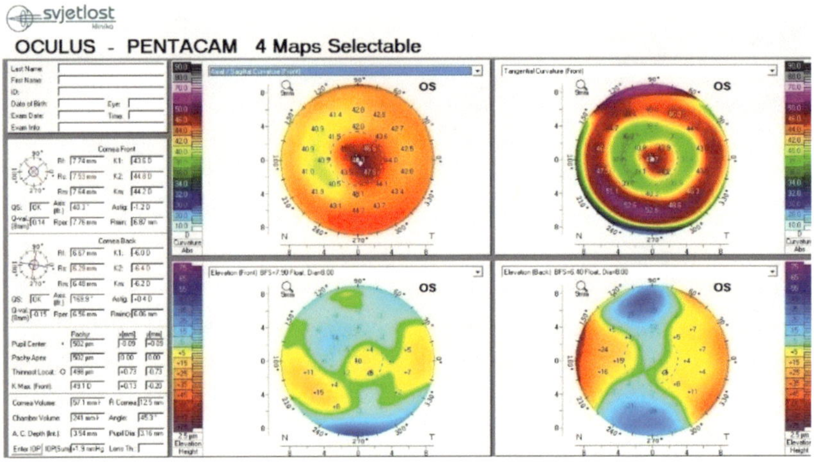

Figure 4.
Central island in patient with buttonhole flap.

2.2.4 General introperative complications

2.2.4.1 Epithelial defect

Epithelial defects are usually caused by the passage of microkeratome over the dry corneal surface or over the epithelium loosened by excessive use of anesthetic drops prior to surgery. Also, a higher risk occurs in patients with history of recurrent erosions, epithelial basement membrane dystrophy (EBDM), drying of the flap, and iatrogenic trauma with surgical instruments [34, 35]. Epithelial defect can be accompanied by stromal oedema and inadequate flap adherence, which increases the risk of inflammatory response as DLK, even epithelial ingrowth [36].

What shall we do?

In case of smaller epithelial defects, frequent use of artificial tears, preferably conservative-free postoperatively is recommended with higher dose of topical corticosteroids in the next few postoperative days, primarily to prevent development of DLK. For larger defects (3 or more mm) bandage soft contact lens needs to be applied to ensure smooth epithelial healing.

2.2.4.2 Interface debris

Interlamellar contamination (debris) may consist of connective and skin epithelial cells, Meibomian gland secretions, talc from the gloves, sponge fibers, metallic particles from microkeratome, and eyelash [4] (**Figure 5**). Interface debris should be carefully differentiated from an infectious or inflammatory reaction. However, impurities can support infectious or sterile inflammation of the cornea and cause mechanical disturbances in vision when placed on the visual axis [1, 37].

What should we do?

In most cases, debris does not induce inflammation since it is biodegradable, but it should be observed. However, if there is any suspicion of an inflammatory reaction or large amount of debris covering the visual axis, causing significant visual disturbances, it should be managed with flap lift and thorough irrigation [38].

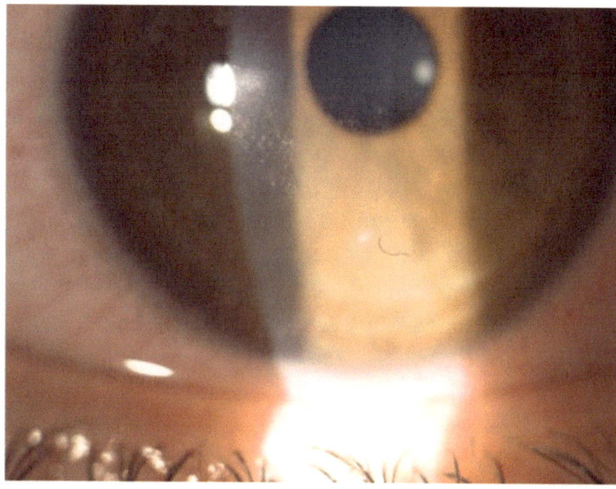

Figure 5.
Interface debris visible at 1st postoperative day.

2.3 Postoperative complications

2.3.1 Early postoperative complications

2.3.1.1 Flap striae

Flap striae occur in 0.03–3.5%, according to the literature [39] and are usually observed the next day after the surgery at the slit-lamp examination, best in retroillumination or with fluorescein staining at cobalt-blue light (**Figure 6**). In cases where flap is edematous, epithelial microstriae can present within 7 days postoperatively. Striae can be classified as micro- and macrostriae. Microstriae are irregularities in epithelial layer, where macrostriae result as full-thickness flap-folds. AT higher risk are cases with high refractive error ("tenting" effect due to the flap and stromal bed

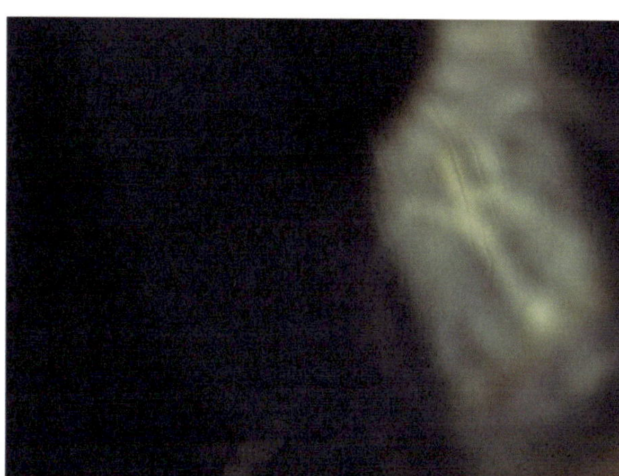

Figure 6.
Vertical flap striae at 1st postoperative day without flap dislocation.

contour mismatch), misalignment during repositioning, excessive manipulation of the flap during surgery, and flap contracture [3, 4, 40].

What shall we do?

Flap striae involving visual axis (inducing irregular astigmatism and optical aberrations) should be treated. When microstriae are presented early after the surgery, gentle stroking in a perpendicular way (flap sliding technique) with wet surgical sponge is sufficient [41]. Macrostriae must be managed with flap re-lift, stroking with surgical sponge on both stromal and epithelial side of the flap, and then careful flap repositioning. Fixed striae and flap-folds often present with epithelial hyperplasia, therefore epithelium and stromal bed debridement are necessary along with flap lift, repositioning, and stroking.

2.3.1.2 Flap dislocation

Dislocation of the flap most commonly occurs in the first 24 hours after surgery before epithelial healing of the lamellar incision occurs (**Figure 7**). However, dislocations are possible several months after the procedure, usually after ocular trauma (**Figure 8**). Flap dislocation is considered an emergency and should be treated immediately to prevent folds and epithelial ingrowth. Patients present with sudden onset blurred vision, often associated with pain in the early postoperative period, the most common cause is mechanical due to lid squeezing, forceful blinking, and rubbing of eyes. Larger diameter flaps, thinner, and those with a small hinge are more susceptible to movement. In some cases, after repositioning the flap, DLK, interface haze, or epithelial ingrowth can occur [1, 42, 43].

What shall we do?

Dislodged flap needs to be managed with flap lift, debridement of stromal bed and stromal side of the flap for possible epithelium (preventing ingrowth), interface irrigation, and flap repositioning. Careful flap handling, soft stroking, and meticulous edge drying are of great importance. BSCL is often applied, and patient is rechecked after half an hour to confirm the flap position and edge adherence [35, 44].

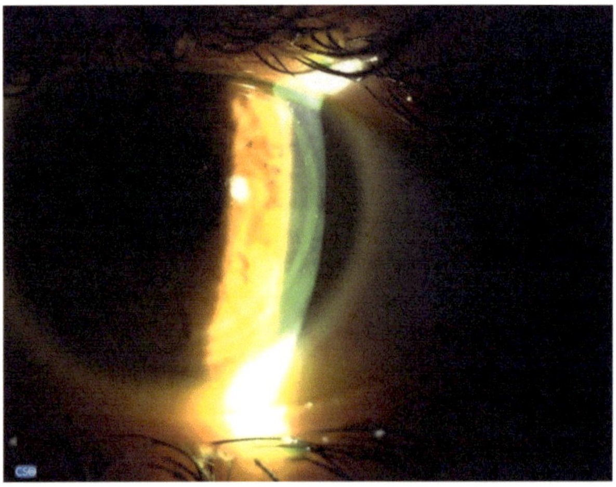

Figure 7.
Dislodged flap due with associated vertical striae due to eye rubbing at 1st postoperative day.

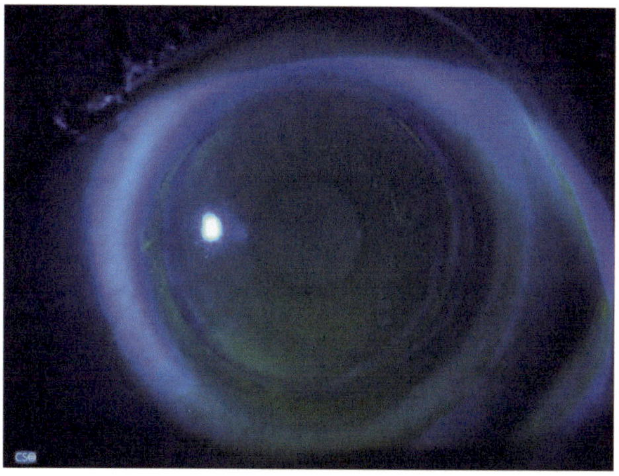

Figure 8.
Late flap dislocation 3 months after LASIK procedure due to blunt eye trauma. Patient presented 2 hours after the trauma occurred.

2.3.1.3 Residual refractive error (under- or overcorrection)

Residual refractive error has been reported in up to 50% of LASIK cases [45]. Hypocorrection is the most common complication after primary LASIK and is usually diagnosed within the first few weeks after surgery. Hypercorrections are more common after repeated procedures and in elderly patients due to slightly dehydrated cornea (>50 years). Hypo- and hypercorrections are associated with excimer laser ablation algorithm, inaccurate nomograms, age, height of refractive error [45–48], and even environmental factors can affect the amount of tissue ablation depth (temperature, humidity, and atmospheric pressure) [49]. Additionally, cyclotorsion from erect to supine position and poor centration of eye during laser ablation can cause postoperative astigmatism [50].

What shall we do?

After confirmed refractive and topography stabilization, re-lift with LASIK or PRK enhancement can be done. There is a slight risk of epithelial defects postoperatively and epithelial ingrowth in case of flap re-lift [45, 51].

2.3.1.4 Diffuse lamellar keratitis (DLK)

Diffuse lamellar keratitis (DLK) is a diffuse sterile inflammation of the lamella between the flap and the stroma (interface). It has been reported in 0.13% to 18.9% of cases [52, 53]. Inflammation may occur within 24 hours or be delayed for several days after the procedure. The course of inflammation is variable, it is possible to gradually reduce, increase or persist the inflammation. Etiological DLK is an allergic or toxic reaction caused by debris left in the lamellae—tears, mucus, corneal epithelial cells, connective tissue or skin, Meibomian gland secretion, glove powder, metal particles or wax from knives, leukocytes or blood from the pannus. An immune response to a temperature-resistant toxin from a sterilizer is also possible [36, 54–59].

Another etiology of DLK is related to the use of femtosecond lasers and photodisruption caused by microscopic tissue injury enhanced by inflammatory mediators from the surface of the eye. DLK was much more common in older models of femtosecond high-energy lasers. Today, only mild transient lamellar keratitis is seen on the periphery of the flap associated with slightly higher energies required for the formation of lateral incisions [36, 58, 59].

Symptoms include discomfort, mild to moderate pain, foreign body sensation, tearing, and light-scattering, A typical lamellar infiltrate is composed of white granular opacities limited to the lamella, without epithelial defects and reactions in the anterior chamber, while conjunctival injection can be present. DLK is divided into four stages or degrees by Linebarger et al. (I degree mild, IV degree melting of the flap) for the purpose of appropriate treatment in a timely manner and prognosis (**Figures 9** and **10**) [1, 60].

What shall we do?

When presented at grade 1 or 2, an intensive topical steroid is necessary and recheck within next 24–48 hours is crucial for early identification of cases progressing to grade 3. Early flap lift and irrigation of interface with intensive topical steroids in grade 3 should reduce the risk of progression to stage 4. There are some recommendations for introducing peroral Doxycycline in addition to standard treatment regime for advanced grades. Even though, usually there is no major benefit of any intervention after progression to grade 4 [60].

2.3.1.5 Central toxic keratopathy (CTK)

CTK is a rare acute, non-inflammatory central corneal opacification that occurs within days of uncomplicated LASIK or PRK. Incidence is reported in 0.02%–0.016% of cases [61, 62], and the etiology is unknown, but enzymatic degradation of keratocytes is suspected. Activated keratocytes without inflammatory cells with initial loss of stromal keratocytes and subsequent gradual repopulation were found by confocal microscopy. CTK causes central corneal haze, (**Figure 11**), thinning of corneal stroma, and flattening of the anterior corneal surface, mostly without affecting the posterior surface. It is important to differentiate it diagnostically from stage IV DLK. Unlike DLK, CTK develops acute within 3–9 days postoperatively as central opacification, rarely associated with conjunctival hyperemia, or ciliary flush.

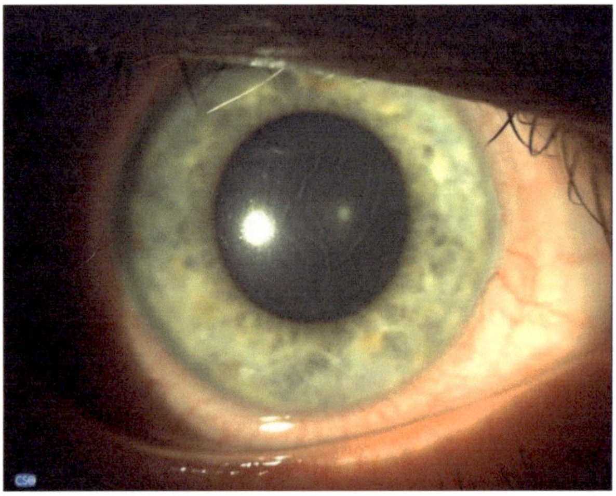

Figure 9.
DLK at grade II, inflammatory reaction visible throughout complete interface, without signs of melting.

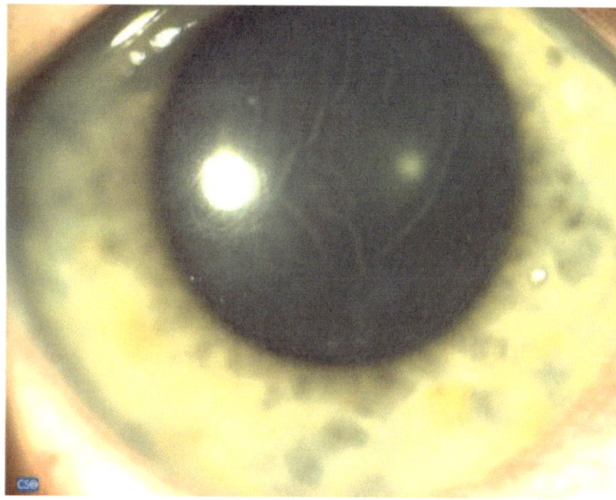

Figure 10.
DLK in advanced grade, visible inflammatory reaction forming characteristic shifting sands phenomenon "sands of Sahara".

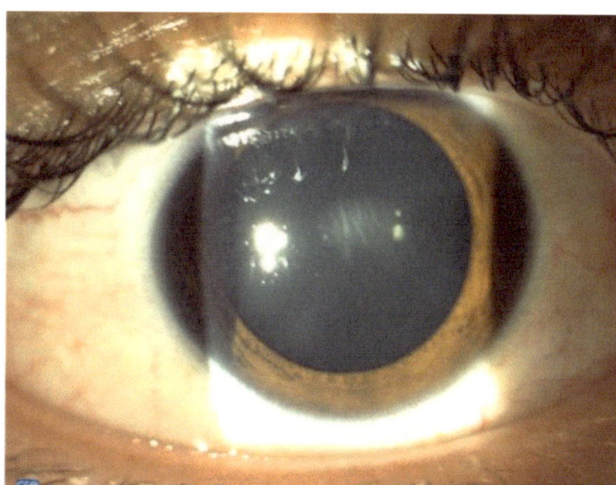

Figure 11.
Central toxic keratopathy in patient presented 5 days after LASIK procedure. Visible centralized opacification that extends anteriorly or posteriorly from the interface.

What shall we do?

Since CTK is a non-inflammatory condition, steroids are not indicated, thus they may hamper the healing process. Usually, there is spontaneous recovery without specific therapy needed. Recovery phase takes up to 18 months, where slight central opacification can remain, but corneal thickness increases and hyperopic shift decreases [61, 63–66].

2.3.1.6 Pressure-induced stromal keratitis

PISK, also known as interface fluid syndrome [67] is a relatively rapid response to corticosteroids that presents with elevated intraocular pressure and fluid accumulation in the lamella between the flap and the adjacent corneal stroma. The amount of fluid varies and can be very small and clinically present as diffuse stroma opacity or large, clinically clearly separating the flap from the adjacent stroma. PISK is often misdiagnosed with DLK, bud the main difference is occurrence at least 5–7 days postoperatively, with high IOP and poor response to corticosteroids, au contraire. Hence, it is extremely important to differentiate it diagnostically from DLK in order to discontinue corticosteroid therapy. The values of intraocular pressure due to fluid are centrally falsely low, while peripheral measurements show somewhat more accurate results [63, 68].

What shall we do?

Management includes cessation of corticosteroid therapy and introduction of anti-glaucoma therapy for avoiding glaucomatous optic nerve damage [69, 70].

2.3.1.7 Infectious keratitis

Infectious keratitis is a rare but potentially devastating and sight-threatening complication after LASIK. It is rare, with 0.034–0.2% cases with decreased incidence over the years [71, 72]. It can be caused by viruses (Adenoviruses, Herpes simplex virus), bacteria (Staphylococcus, Pseudomonas), atypical mycobacteria, fungi, and parasites (Acanthamoeba). Infectious keratitis is divided into early (within the first two postoperative weeks) and late (occurs 2–3 months after surgery). Early infectious keratitis is caused by staphylococci and streptococci (most often methicillin-resistant staphylococci), and late atypical mycobacteria and fungi. The risk of infection is blepharitis, dry eye, intraoperative epithelial defects, intraoperative contamination, prolonged epithelialization after surgery, and certain professions (medical professionals). Symptoms may include pain, lightheadedness, tearing, decreased visual acuity, image duplication, shadows, and haloes. Examination on a biomicroscope may show ciliary injection, epithelial defects, anterior chamber reaction, and hypopion. Fungal keratitis, although significantly rarer than bacterial, should be considered in the differential diagnosis [1, 73–76].

What shall we do?

When it comes to infectious keratitis, prophylaxis is preferred over treatment. Proper use of sterile gloves, caps, instruments, and betadine wash of eyelids prior to the surgery will reduce the risk of infection. In observed infectious keratitis, management includes flap lift, scraping of bed, and irrigation of bed with antibiotics. In early onset, the best choice is vancomycin and amikacin in late-onset. Cessation of corticosteroids is obligatory, and topical fourth-generation fluoroquinolone and vancomycin (early onset) or amikacin with vancomycin 5% or topical clarithromycin and 4th generation fluoroquinolone for late-onset [72]. After culture isolation and the accompanying sensitivity antibiogram, local antibiotic therapy is revised. Sometimes, in case of severe infection, flap amputation is needed, both for therapeutic and diagnostic reasons [73].

2.3.1.8 Stromal melting or flap melting

Stromal melting is mostly unilateral and occurs 2–5 weeks after LASIK. It most commonly occurs after epithelial defects, thin and/or irregular flaps, perforated flaps, epithelial ingrowth, and deep lamellar keratitis. It may also be associated with systemic immune diseases such as thyroiditis, systemic lupus, Sjögren's disease, rheumatoid arthritis, eczema, and erythema. The disease is usually self-limiting for 21–45 days and results in variable intensity of opacification (leukemia) and regular or incorrect astigmatism. Melting of the flap is very likely caused by apoptosis induced by an implanted layer of epithelial cells caused by epithelial ingrowth. Epithelial ingrowth, as well as possible melting of the flap edge, is more common in reoperations, especially in hyperopic eyes, than in primary operations [77–79].

2.3.1.9 Transient photosensitivity

It is characterized by light-headedness and mild pain with normal visual acuity but without inflammation. It occurs a few days after the procedure and can last for several weeks. The complication is related to the high energy and low frequency of mostly older generations of femtosecond lasers, and the hypothetical cause is the stimulation of keratocytes and corneal nerves by the shock waves of the femtosecond laser [80].

2.3.2 Late postoperative complications

2.3.2.1 Refractive regression

Regression is the return of diopters in the direction of primary refractive error documented in several arrivals 3–6 months after LASIK. Regression is more common after hyperopic LASIK, observed in nearly 30% of hyperopes and 5.5–27.7% of myopes [81]. Regression after LASIK is associated with an increase in corneal thickness and curvature. Potential mechanisms involved in regression include nucleus sclerosis, stromal synthesis and remodeling (wound healing), compensatory epithelial hyperplasia, decreased flap thickness, an anterior shift of cornea, and iatrogenic keratectasia [82].

What shall we do?

After confirmed refractive stability, within 3–4 months, enhancement with LASIK re-lift, PRK, or even LASEK can be advised.

2.3.2.2 Epithelial ingrowth

Epithelial ingrowth at the terminal periphery of the flap is normal flap healing. Clinically significant epithelial ingrowth occurs when a fistula develops under the flap, which allows epithelial cells to migrate in the lamella between the flap and the stroma and causes opacification. It occurs in 0−3.9% of cases undergoing primary treatment and 10−20% in re-treatment cases [83]. In primary uncomplicated LASIK, a higher incidence of epithelial ingrowth was observed in the treatment of hyperopia, in microkeratome compared to femtosecond lasers, LASIK after radial keratotomy, intraoperative epithelial defects, and in the elderly. After repeated procedures and application of therapeutic soft contact lenses, an increased incidence of epithelial ingrowth was observed, as well as in operations performed three or more years after primary LASIK. Isolated epithelial islets rarely cause problems (**Figure 12**). However, if the ingrowth is connected to the superficial epithelium and continues to grow and reach the visual axis, it can cause distortion of the flap surface and the development of irregular astigmatism (**Figure 13**). Symptoms of epithelial ingrowth include light-headedness, glare, decreased visual acuity, and foreign body sensation. Theoretically, there are several ways in which epithelial cells can get into the lamella: by mechanical indentation on the microkeratome blade or with water during irrigation after photoablation, and by ingrowth of cells derived from peripheral epithelium.

Biomicroscopically, epithelial ingrowth is shown with epithelial beads in the lamella formed by dividing epithelial cells, fluorescein accumulation at the edges of

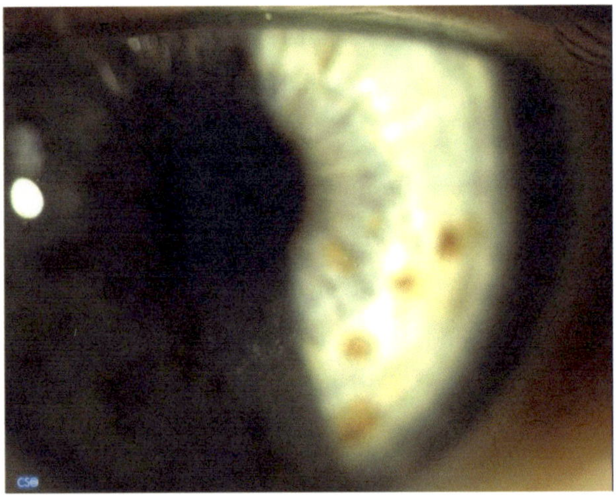

Figure 12.
Epithelial cell collection under the flap.

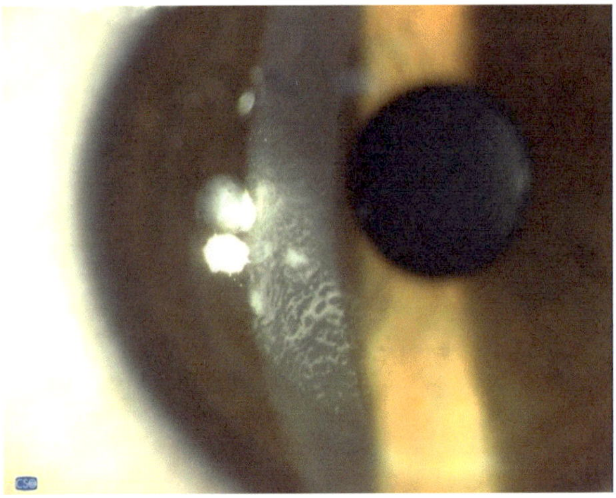

Figure 13.
Epithelial ingrowth from flap margin advancing to the central part of the interface.

the flap or even below the flap, fibrotic demarcation line at the leading edge of epithelial ingrowth, keratolysis, or melting of the flap edge [63, 84–87]. Patients usually present with foreign body sensation and dysphotopsia (glare) in the early stages and decreased visual acuity in later stages.

What shall we do?

In the initial stages (grade 1) observation is recommended, but for advanced stages, flap lift, thorough mechanical debridement of epithelial cells with profound wash of stromal bed, and Mitomycine C 0.02% application for preventing ingrowth recurrence (observed in one-third of cases) [83]. Some literature advise low energy (0.6 mJ) Nd-YAG laser for treating ingrowth [83, 88].

2.3.2.3 Induced and iatrogenic keratectasia

Iatrogenic keratectasia is a serious complication seen in 0.033–0.6% cases [4, 89] associated with a weakening of the mechanical strength of the cornea. It is clinically presented by progressive weakening of uncorrected visual acuity and increase in myopia, and by progressive increase in corneal curvature visible on corneal topography (**Figure 14**). Iatrogenic keratectasia occurs several weeks to several years after the procedure. The flap does not contribute to the biomechanical strength of the cornea, and all biomechanical stress is tolerated by untreated deeper parts of the cornea. Risk factors include irregular corneal topography, thin central corneal thickness (<450 μm), low residual corneal thickness (<250 μm), young age, and high spherical refractive error equivalent [90–92].

What shall we do?

In the case of keratectasia, prophylaxis as careful and detailed screening of corneal topography is of most importance. When progressive ectasia is observed, collagen Cross-linking is performed. Additionally, rigid gas-permeable CL or intracorneal ring segments can restore vision. For advanced cases, anterior lamellar keratoplasty or event perforative keratoplasty is required [89, 93].

2.3.2.4 Dry eye

Corneal refractive surgery can induce or even worsen dry eye symptoms (**Figure 15**). Dry eye syndrome causes discomfort, fluctuations in vision quality, delayed healing and epithelial damage, and can lead to regression of refractive error and reduced vision quality. In most patients, the symptoms are mild and do not cause interference, and pass within 6 months when the healing period ends. According to the literature and clinical practice, dry eye is observed in more than 90% of cases [94]. The main risk factors for chronic dry eye after surgery are preoperative dry eye and female sex [95–98]. Symptoms of dry eye are thought to be caused by denervation and cutting of nerve fibers during flap formation,

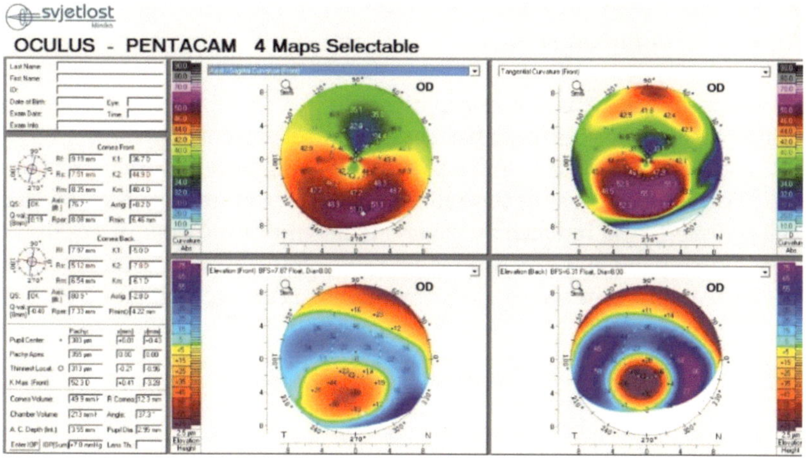

Figure 14.
Iatrogenic corneal ectasia 1 year after LASIK procedure.

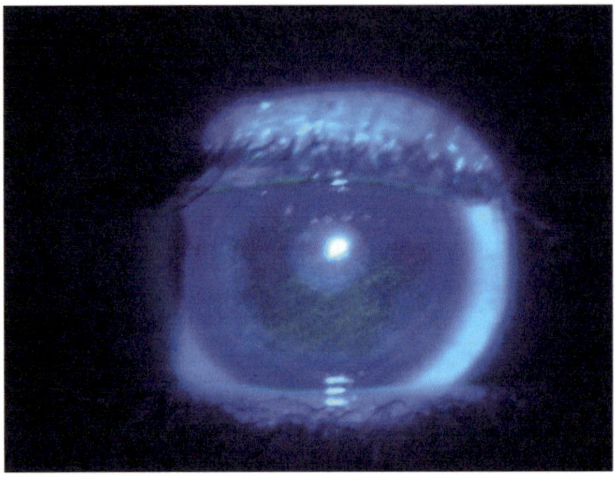

Figure 15.
Severe dry eye 1 month after LASIK procedure.

excimer laser removal of corneal tissue, and corneal reshaping. Denervation causes a decrease in corneal sensitivity and interrupts the flow of information from the cornea to the lacrimal system. Lack of corneal sensitivity can lead to a decrease in the number of blinks, and to a lack of information about the need to produce a larger amount and/or a specific tear component. Improvement in corneal sensation and DED by 3–6 months occur in most cases, but corneal innervation can be delayed by 2–3 years [99].

What shall we do?

The choice of patients and the treatment of dry eye symptoms before the procedure are extremely important. Standard therapy includes artificial tears for prolonged period of 6 months or longer, and topical corticosteroids (currently most commonly used is low dose hydrocortisone) [100]. In severe cases of DED, topical cyclosporine drops and Punctal Plug instillation for occluding tear punctum.

2.3.2.5 Night vision disturbances

The main cause of decreased vision quality and glare symptoms is an increase in spherical aberration in the centrally flattened cornea. Symptoms worsen at night due to the physiological dilation of the pupil and the entry of light rays through the untreated periphery. Glare can also cause decentralized ablations, too small optical zones, newly formed lens blurring, and induced astigmatism. Patients with scotopic pupils larger than 7.5 mm and high myopic corrections are most often affected. Fortunately, most symptoms resolve over time without treatment due to cortical adaptation [101–104].

3. Conclusions

It is of the greatest interest for every refractive surgeon to perform safe surgery and successfully treat possible complications. Therefore, meticulous knowledge of intraoperative and postoperative complications will ensure timely and appropriate preventive measures to reduce the occurrence of complications, their early detection, and appropriate management in order to achieve optimal results.

Conflict of interest

The authors declare no conflict of interest.

Author details

Fanka Gilevska[1], Maja Bohač[2], Smiljka Popović Suić[2] and Mateja Jagić[2]*

1 Eye Clinic Sistina Oftalmologija, North Macedonia

2 University Eye Clinic Svjetlost, Croatia

*Address all correspondence to: mateja.jagic@svjetlost.hr

References

[1] Farah SG, Ghanem RC, Azar DT. LASIK complications and their management. In: Azar DT, editor. Refractive Surgery. 2nd ed. Philadelphia: Elsevier Inc; 2007. pp. 195-221. DOI:10.1016/B978-0-323-03599-6.50076-6

[2] Vayr F, Chastang P, Hoang-Xuan T. Laser and mechanical microkeratomes. In: Azar DT, editor. Refractive Surgery. 2nd. ed. Philadelphia: Elsevier Inc; 2007. pp. 147-155. DOI: 10.1016/B978-0-323-03599-6.50072-9

[3] Moshirfar M, Gardiner JP, Schliesser JA, et al. Laser in situ keratomileusis flap complications using mechanical microkeratome versus femtosecond laser: Retrospective comparison. Journal of Cataract and Refractive Surgery. 2010;**36**(11):1925-1933. DOI: 10.1016/j.jcrs.2010.05.027

[4] Melki SA, Azar DT. LASIK complications: Etiology, management, and prevention. Survey of Ophthalmology. 2001;**46**(2):95-116. DOI: 10.1016/s0039-6257(01)00254-5

[5] Rao SK, Padmanabhan P, Sitalakshmi G, Rajagopal R. Partial flap during laser in-situ keratomileusis: Pathogenesis and timing of retreatment. Indian Journal of Ophthalmology. 2000;**48**(3):209-212

[6] Jain V, Mhatre K, Shome D. Flap buttonhole in thin-flap laser in situ keratomileusis: Case series and review. Cornea. 2010;**29**(6):655-658. DOI: 10.1097/ICO.0b013e3181c377d5

[7] Leung AT, Rao SK, Cheng AC, Yu EW, Fan DS, Lam DS. Pathogenesis and management of laser in situ keratomileusis flap buttonhole. Journal of Cataract and Refractive Surgery. 2000;**26**(3):358-362. DOI: 10.1016/s0886-3350(99)00414-9

[8] Tham VM, Maloney RK. Microkeratome complications of laser in situ keratomileusis. Ophthalmology. 2000;**107**(5):920-924. DOI: 10.1016/s0161-6420(00)00004-x

[9] Al-Mezaine HS, Al-Amro SA, Al-Obeidan S. Incidence, management, and visual outcomes of buttonholed laser in situ keratomileusis flaps. Journal of Cataract and Refractive Surgery. 2009;**35**(5):839-845. DOI: 10.1016/j.jcrs.2009.01.013

[10] Geggel HS. Treatment of lost flaps and slipped flaps. International Ophthalmology Clinics. 2008;**48**(1):65-71. DOI: 10.1097/IIO.0b013e31815eb96d244

[11] Joo CK, Kim TG. Corneal perforation during laser in situ keratomileusis. Journal of Cataract and Refractive Surgery. 1999;**25**(8):1165-1167. DOI: 10.1016/s0886-3350(99)00117-0

[12] Liu Q, Gong XM, Chen JQ, Yang B, Ge J, To CH. Laser in situ keratomileusis induced corneal perforation and recurrent corneal epithelial ingrowth. Journal of Cataract and Refractive Surgery. 2005;**31**(4):857-859. DOI: 10.1016/j.jcrs.2004.09.027 251

[13] Walton OB, Slade SG. Thin, irregular, buttoonhole flaps. In: Jl A, Azar DT, editors. Management of Complications in Refractive Surgery. Springer Inc.; 2018. pp. 23-26. DOI: 10.1007/978-3-319-60561-6_3

[14] Chung SH, Mazur E. Surgical applications of femtosecond lasers. Journal of Biophotonics.

2009;**2**(10):557-572. DOI: 10.1002/jbio.200910053

[15] Salomão MQ, Wilson SE. Femtosecond laser in laser in situ keratomileusis. Journal of Cataract and Refractive Surgery. 2010;**36**(6):1024-1032. DOI: 10.1016/j.jcrs.2010.03.025

[16] Kymionis GD, Kankariya VP, Plaka AD, Reinstein DZ. Femtosecond laser technology in corneal refractive surgery: A review. Journal of Refractive Surgery. 2012;**28**(12):912-920. DOI: 10.3928/1081597X-20121116-01

[17] Srinivasan S, Rootman DS. Anterior chamber gas bubble formation during femtosecond laser flap creation for LASIK. Journal of Refractive Surgery. 2007;**23**(8):828-830. DOI: 10.3928/1081-597X-20071001-14

[18] Jung HG, Kim J, Lim TH. Possible risk factors and clinical effects of an opaque bubble layer created with femtosecond laser-assisted laser in situ keratomileusis. Journal of Cataract and Refractive Surgery. 2015;**41**(7):1393-1399. DOI: 10.1016/j.jcrs.2014.10.039

[19] Lim DH, Hyun J, Shin E, Ko BW, Chung ES, Chung TY. Incidence and risk factors of opaque bubble layer formation according to flap thickness during 500-kHz FS-LASIK. Journal of Refractive Surgery. 2019;**35**(9):583-589. DOI: 10.3928/1081597X-20190814-01

[20] Hurmeric V, Yoo SH, Fishler J, Chang VS, Wang J, Culbertson WW. In vivo structural characteristics of the femtosecond LASIK-induced opaque bubble layers with ultrahigh-resolution SD-OCT. Ophthalmic Surgery, Lasers & Imaging. 2010;**41**(Suppl.):S109-S113. DOI: 10.3928/15428877-20101031-08

[21] Kanellopoulos AJ, Asimellis G. Digital analysis of flap parameter accuracy and objective assessment of opaque bubble layer in femtosecond laser-assisted LASIK: A novel technique. Clinical Ophthalmology. 2013;7:343-351. DOI: 10.2147/OPTH.S39644

[22] Soong HK, de Melo Franco R. Anterior chamber gas bubbles during femtosecond laser flap creation in LASIK: Video evidence of entry via trabecular meshwork. Journal of Cataract & Refractive Surgery. Dec 2012;**38**(12):2184-2185. DOI: 10.1016/j.jcrs.2012.09.012. Epub 2012 Oct 13. PMID: 23073481

[23] dos Santos AM, Torricelli AA, Marino GK, et al. Femtosecond laser-assisted LASIK flap complications. Journal of Refractive Surgery. 2016;**32**(1):52-59. DOI: 10.3928/1081597X-20151119-01

[24] Tse SM, Farley ND, Tomasko KR, Amin SR. Intraoperative LASIK complications. International Ophthalmology Clinics. 2016;**56**(2):47-57. DOI: 10.1097/IIO.0000000000000110

[25] Srinivasan S, Herzig S. Sub-epithelial gas breakthrough during femtosecond laser flap creation for LASIK. The British Journal of Ophthalmology. 2007;**91**(10):1373. DOI: 10.1136/bjo.2007.129213

[26] Wei CH, Mei LX, Ge Y, Zhang PF. Managements of vertical gas breakthrough in femtosecond laser assisted LASIK. International Journal of Ophthalmology. 2020;**13**(9):1503-1504. DOI: 10.18240/ijo.2020.09.25

[27] Vinciguerra P, Camesasca FI. Decentration after refractive surgery. Journal of Refractive Surgery. 2001;**17**(Suppl. 2):S190-S191. DOI: 10.3928/1081-597X-20010302-07

[28] Melki SA, Azar DT. Eight pearls in prevention and management of LASIK

complications. In: Melki SA, Azar DT, editors. 101 Pearls in Refractive, Cataract and Corneal Surgery. Thorofare, NJ: Slack; 2001. pp. 23-32

[29] Manche E, Roe J. Recent advances in wavefront-guided LASIK. Current Opinion in Ophthalmology. 2018;**29**(4):286-291. DOI: 10.1097/ICU.0000000000000488

[30] Duffey RJ. Central islands and decentered ablations after LASIK. International Ophthalmology Clinics. 2000;**40**(3):93-101. DOI: 10.1097/00004397-200007000-00012

[31] Kang SW, Chung ES, Kim WJ. Clinical analysis of central islands after laser in situ keratomileusis. Journal of Cataract and Refractive Surgery. 2000;**26**(4):536-542. DOI: 10.1016/s0886-3350(99)00458-7

[32] Tsai YY, Lin JM. Natural history of central islands after laser in situ keratomileusis. Journal of Cataract and Refractive Surgery. 2000;**26**(6):853-858. DOI: 10.1016/s0886-3350(00)00375-8

[33] Johnson JD, Azar DT. Surgically induced topographical abnormalities after LASIK: Management of central islands, corneal ectasia, decentration, and irregular astigmatism. Current Opinion in Ophthalmology. 2001;**12**(4):309-317. DOI: 10.1097/00055735-200108000-00012

[34] Randleman JB, Lynn MJ, Banning CS, Stulting RD. Risk factors for epithelial defect formation during laser in situ keratomileusis. Journal of Cataract and Refractive Surgery. 2007;**33**(10):1738-1743. DOI: 10.1016/j.jcrs.2007.05.038

[35] Smirennaia E, Sheludchenko V, Kourenkova N, Kashnikova O. Management of corneal epithelial defects following laser in situ keratomileusis. Journal of Refractive Surgery. 2001;**17**(Suppl. 2):S196-S199. DOI: 10.3928/1081-597X-20010302-09

[36] Shah MN, Misra M, Wihelmus KR, Koch DD. Diffuse lamellar keratitis associated with epithelial defects after laser in situ keratomileusis. Journal of Cataract and Refractive Surgery. 2000;**26**(9):1312-1318. DOI: 10.1016/s0886-3350(00)00570-8

[37] Hirst LW, Vandeleur KW Jr. Laser in situ keratomileusis interface deposits. Journal of Refractive Surgery. 1998;**14**(6):653-654. DOI: 10.3928/1081-597X-19981101-15

[38] Mimouni M, Vainer I, Assad N, et al. Incidence, indications, and outcomes of eyes needing early flap lifting after LASIK. Cornea. 2018;**37**(9):1118-1123. DOI: 10.1097/ICO.0000000000001617

[39] Wallerstein A, Gauvin M, Adiguzel E, et al. Clinically significant laser in situ keratomileusis flap striae. Journal of Cataract and Refractive Surgery. 2017;**43**(12):1523-1533. DOI: 10.1016/j.jcrs.2017.09.023

[40] Shah DN, Melki S. Complications of femtosecond-assisted laser in-situ keratomileusis flaps. Seminars in Ophthalmology. 2014;**29**(5-6):363-375. DOI: 10.3109/08820538.2014.959194

[41] Abdelazeem K, Nassr MA, Abdelmotaal H, Wasfi E, El-Sebaity DM. Flap sliding technique for managing flap striae following laser in situ keratomileusis. Journal of Ophthalmology. 2020;**2020**:5614327. [Accessed: February 24, 2020]. DOI: 10.1155/2020/5614327

[42] Hardten DR, Hardten AG, Hardten SA. Management of the distorted Flap. In: Alio J, Azar D, editors. Management of Complications

in Refractive Surgery. Cham: Springer; 2018. pp. 33-36. DOI: 10.1007/978-3-319-60561-6_5

[43] Iskander NG, Peters NT, Anderson Penno E, Gimbel HV. Late traumatic flap dislocation after laser in situ keratomileusis. Journal of Cataract and Refractive Surgery. 2001;**27**(7):1111-1114. DOI: 10.1016/s0886-3350(01)00752-0

[44] Clare G, Moore TC, Grills C, Leccisotti A, Moore JE, Schallhorn S. Early flap displacement after LASIK. Ophthalmology. 2011;**118**(9):1760-1765. DOI: 10.1016/j.ophtha.2011.01.053

[45] Netto MV, Wilson SE. Flap lift for LASIK retreatment in eyes with myopia. Ophthalmology. 2004;**111**(7):1362-1367. DOI: 10.1016/j.ophtha.2003.11.009

[46] Yuen LH, Chan WK, Koh J, Mehta JS, Tan DT. SingLasik research group. A 10-year prospective audit of LASIK outcomes for myopia in 37,932 eyes at a single institution in Asia. Ophthalmology. 2010;**117**(6):1236-1244. e1. DOI: 10.1016/j.ophtha.2009.10.042

[47] Alió JL, Muftuoglu O, Ortiz D, et al. Ten-year follow-up of laser in situ keratomileusis for myopia of up to −10 diopters. American Journal of Ophthalmology. 2008;**145**(1):46-54. DOI: 10.1016/j.ajo.2007.09.010

[48] Randleman JB, White AJ Jr, Lynn MJ, Hu MH, Stulting RD. Incidence, outcomes, and risk factors for retreatment after wavefront-optimized ablations with PRK and LASIK. Journal of Refractive Surgery. 2009;**25**(3):273-276. DOI: 10.3928/1081597X-20090301-06 62

[49] Hood CT, Shtein RM, Veldheer D, et al. The effect of humidity and temperature on visual outcomes after myopic corneal laser refractive surgery. Clinical Ophthalmology. 2016;**10**:2231-2236. [Accessed: November 4, 2016]. DOI: 10.2147/OPTH.S118503

[50] Shen EP, Chen WL, Hu FR. Manual limbal markings versus iris-registration software for correction of myopic astigmatism by laser in situ keratomileusis. Journal of Cataract and Refractive Surgery. 2010;**36**(3):431-436. DOI: 10.1016/j.jcrs.2009.10.030

[51] Schallhorn SC, Venter JA, Hannan SJ, Hettinger KA, Teenan D. Flap lift and photorefractive keratectomy enhancements after primary laser in situ keratomileusis using a wavefront-guided ablation profile: Refractive and visual outcomes. Journal of Cataract and Refractive Surgery. 2015;**41**(11):2501-2512. DOI: 10.1016/j.jcrs.2015.05.031

[52] Gritz DC. LASIK interface keratitis: Epidemiology, diagnosis and care. Current Opinion in Ophthalmology. 2011;**22**(4):251-255. DOI: 10.1097/ICU.0b013e3283477b52

[53] Smith RJ, Maloney RK. Diffuse lamellar keratitis. A new syndrome in lamellar refractive surgery. Ophthalmology. 1998;**105**(9):1721-1726. DOI: 10.1016/S0161-6420(98)99044-3

[54] MacRae S, Macaluso DC, Rich LF. Sterile interface keratitis associated with micropannus hemorrhage after laser in situ keratomileusis. Journal of Cataract and Refractive Surgery. 1999;**25**(12):1679-1681. DOI: 10.1016/s0886-3350(99)00248-5

[55] Holland SP, Mathias RG, Morck DW, Chiu J, Slade SG. Diffuse lamellar keratitis related to endotoxins released from sterilizer reservoir biofilms. Ophthalmology. 2000;**107**(7):1227-1234. DOI: 10.1016/s0161-6420(00)00246-3

[56] Kaufman SC. Post-LASIK interface keratitis, Sands of the Sahara syndrome,

and microkeratome blades. Journal of Cataract and Refractive Surgery. 1999;**25**(5):603-604

[57] Fogla R, Rao SK, Padmanabhan P. Diffuse lamellar keratitis: Are meibomian secretions responsible? Journal of Cataract and Refractive Surgery. 2001;**27**(4):493-495. DOI: 10.1016/s0886-3350(01)00819-7

[58] Gil-Cazorla R, Teus MA, de Benito-Llopis L, Fuentes I. Incidence of diffuse lamellar keratitis after laser in situ keratomileusis associated with the IntraLase 15 kHz femtosecond laser and Moria M2 microkeratome. Journal of Cataract and Refractive Surgery. 2008;**34**(1):28-31. DOI: 10.1016/j.jcrs.2007.08.025

[59] Choe CH, Guss C, Musch DC, Niziol LM, Shtein RM. Incidence of diffuse lamellar keratitis after LASIK with 15 KHz, 30 KHz, and 60 KHz femtosecond laser flap creation. Journal of Cataract and Refractive Surgery. 2010;**36**(11):1912-1918. DOI: 10.1016/j.jcrs.2010.09.003

[60] Linebarger EJ, Hardten DR, Lindstrom RL. Diffuse lamellar keratitis: Diagnosis and management. Journal of Cataract and Refractive Surgery. 2000;**26**(7):1072-1077. DOI: 10.1016/s0886-3350(00)00468-5

[61] Moshirfar M, Hazin R, Khalifa YM. Central toxic keratopathy. Current Opinion in Ophthalmology. 2010;**21**(4):274-279. DOI: 10.1097/ICU.0b013e32833a8cb2

[62] Jutley G, Aiello F, Robaei D, Maurino V. Central toxic keratopathy after laser in situ keratomileusis. Journal of Cataract and Refractive Surgery. 2014;**40**(12):1985-1993. DOI: 10.1016/j.jcrs.2014.03.030

[63] Randleman JB, Shah RD. LASIK interface complications: Etiology, management, and outcomes. Journal of Refractive Surgery. 2012;**28**(8):575-586. DOI: 10.3928/1081597X-20120722-01

[64] Hazin R, Daoud YJ, Khalifa YM. What is central toxic keratopathy syndrome if it is not diffuse lamellar keratitis grade IV? Middle East African Journal of Ophthalmology. 2010;**17**(1):60-62. DOI: 10.4103/0974-9233.61218

[65] Thornton IL, Foulks GN, Eiferman RA. Confocal microscopy of central toxic keratopathy. Cornea. 2012;**31**(8):934-936. DOI: 10.1097/ICO.0b013e3181f7f109

[66] Sikder S, Khalifa YM, Neuffer MC, Moshirfar M. Tomographic corneal profile analysis of central toxic keratopathy after LASIK. Cornea. 2012;**31**(1):48-51. DOI: 10.1097/ICO.0b013e31821de341

[67] Tourtas T, Kopsachilis N, Meiller R, Kruse FE, Cursiefen C. Pressure-induced interlamellar stromal keratitis after laser in situ keratomileusis. Cornea. 2011;**30**(8):920-923. DOI: 10.1097/ICO.0b013e3182032002

[68] Belin MW, Hannush SB, Yau CW, Schultze RL. Elevated intraocular pressure-induced interlamellar stromal keratitis. Ophthalmology. 2002;**109**(10):1929-1933. DOI: 10.1016/s0161-6420(02)01163-6

[69] Kurian M, Shetty R, Shetty BK, Devi SA. In vivo confocal microscopic findings of interlamellar stromal keratopathy induced by elevated intraocular pressure. Journal of Cataract and Refractive Surgery. 2006;**32**(9):1563-1566. DOI: 10.1016/j.jcrs.2006.03.041

[70] Cabral-Macias J, García-De la Rosa G, Rodríguez-Matilde DF, et al. Pressure-induced stromal keratopathy

after laser in situ keratomileusis: Acute and late-onset presentations. Journal of Cataract and Refractive Surgery. 2018;**44**(10):1284-1290. DOI: 10.1016/j.jcrs.2018.06.053

[71] Ortega-Usobiaga J, Llovet-Osuna F, Djodeyre MR, Llovet-Rausell A, Beltran J, Baviera J. Incidence of corneal infections after laser in situ keratomileusis and surface ablation when moxifloxacin and tobramycin are used as postoperative treatment. Journal of Cataract and Refractive Surgery. 2015;**41**(6):1210-1216

[72] Donnenfeld ED, Kim T, Holland EJ, et al. ASCRS White Paper: Management of infectious keratitis following laser in situ keratomileusis. Journal of Cataract and Refractive Surgery. 2005;**31**(10):2008-2011. DOI: 10.1016/j.jcrs.2005.10.030

[73] Moshirfar M, Welling JD, Feiz V, Holz H, Clinch TE. Infectious and noninfectious keratitis after laser in situ keratomileusis Occurrence, management, and visual outcomes. Journal of Cataract and Refractive Surgery. 2007;**33**(3):474-483. DOI: 10.1016/j.jcrs.2006.11.005

[74] Solomon R, Donnenfeld ED, Azar DT, et al. Infectious keratitis after laser in situ keratomileusis: results of an ASCRS survey. Journal of Cataract and Refractive Surgery. 2003;**29**(10):2001-2006. DOI: 10.1016/s0886-3350(03)00512-1

[75] Solomon R, Donnenfeld ED, Perry HD, et al. Methicillin-resistant Staphylococcus aureus infectious keratitis following refractive surgery. American Journal of Ophthalmology. 2007;**143**(4):629-634. DOI: 10.1016/j.ajo.2006.12.029

[76] Garg P, Chaurasia S, Vaddavalli PK, Muralidhar R, Mittal V, Gopinathan U. Microbial keratitis after LASIK. Journal of Refractive Surgery. 2010;**26**(3):209-216. DOI: 10.3928/1081597X-20100224-07

[77] Güell JL, Morral M, Elies D, Gris O, Gaytan J, Manero F. Melting. In: Alio JL, Azar DT, editors. Management of Complications in Refractive Surgery. 2nd ed. Springer; 2018. pp. 91-98

[78] Castillo A, Diaz-Valle D, Gutierrez AR, Toledano N, Romero F. Peripheral melt of flap after laser in situ keratomileusis. Journal of Refractive Surgery. 1998;**14**(1):61-63. DOI: 10.3928/1081-597X-19980101-12

[79] Smith RJ, Maloney RK. Laser in situ keratomileusis in patients with autoimmune diseases. Journal of Cataract and Refractive Surgery. 2006;**32**(8):1292-1295. DOI: 10.1016/j.jcrs.2006.02.059

[80] Stonecipher KG, Dishler JG, Ignacio TS, Binder PS. Transient light sensitivity after femtosecond laser flap creation: Clinical findings and management. Journal of Cataract and Refractive Surgery. 2006;**32**(1):91-94. DOI: 10.1016/j.jcrs.2005.11.015

[81] Yan MK, Chang JS, Chan TC. Refractive regression after laser in situ keratomileusis. Clinical & Experimental Ophthalmology. 2018;**46**(8):934-944. DOI: 10.1111/ceo.13315

[82] Alió JL, Soria F, Abbouda A, Peña-García P. Laser in situ keratomileusis for −6.00 to −18.00 diopters of myopia and up to −5.00 diopters of astigmatism: 15-year follow-up. Journal of Cataract and Refractive Surgery. 2015;**41**(1):33-40. DOI: 10.1016/j.jcrs.2014.08.029

[83] Ting DSJ, Srinivasan S, Danjoux JP. Epithelial ingrowth following laser in situ keratomileusis (LASIK): Prevalence, risk factors, management and visual

outcomes. BMJ Open Ophthalmology. 2018;**3**(1):e000133. [Accessed: March 29, 2018]. DOI: 10.1136/bmjophth-2017-000133

[84] Chen S, Feng Y, Stojanovic A, Jankov MR 2nd, Wang Q. IntraLase femtosecond laser vs mechanical microkeratomes in LASIK for myopia: A systematic review and meta-analysis. Journal of Refractive Surgery. 2012;**28**(1):15-24. DOI: 10.3928/1081597X-20111228-02

[85] Friehmann A, Mimouni M, Nemet AY, Sela T, Munzer G, Kaiserman I. Risk factors for epithelial ingrowth following microkeratome-assisted LASIK. Journal of Refractive Surgery. 2018;**34**(2):100-105. DOI: 10.3928/1081597X-20180105-01

[86] Asano-Kato N, Toda I, Hori-Komai Y, Takano Y, Tsubota K. Epithelial ingrowth after laser in situ keratomileusis: Clinical features and possible mechanisms. American Journal of Ophthalmology. 2002;**134**(6):801-807. DOI: 10.1016/s0002-9394(02)01757-9

[87] Caster AI, Friess DW, Schwendeman FJ. Incidence of epithelial ingrowth in primary and retreatment laser in situ keratomileusis. Journal of Cataract and Refractive Surgery. 2010;**36**(1):97-101. DOI: 10.1016/j.jcrs.2009.07.039

[88] Mohammed OA, Mounir A, Hassan AA, Alsmman AH, Mostafa EM. Nd:YAG laser for epithelial ingrowth after laser in situ keratomileusis. International Ophthalmology. 2019;**39**(6):1225-1230. DOI: 10.1007/s10792-018-0923-1

[89] Bohac M, Koncarevic M, Pasalic A, et al. Incidence and clinical characteristics of post LASIK Ectasia: A review of over 30,000 LASIK cases. Seminars in Ophthalmology. 2018;**33**(7-8):869-877. DOI: 10.1080/08820538.2018.1539183

[90] Randleman JB, Woodward M, Lynn MJ, Stulting RD. Risk assessment for ectasia after corneal refractive surgery. Ophthalmology. 2008;**115**(1):37-50. DOI: 10.1016/j.ophtha.2007.03.073

[91] Klein SR, Epstein RJ, Randleman JB, Stulting RD. Corneal ectasia after laser in situ keratomileusis in patients without apparent preoperative risk factors. Cornea. 2006;**25**(4):388-403. DOI: 10.1097/01.ico.0000222479.68242.77

[92] Seiler T, Quurke AW. Iatrogenic keratectasia after LASIK in a case of forme fruste keratoconus. Journal of Cataract and Refractive Surgery. 1998;**24**(7):1007-1009. DOI: 10.1016/s0886-3350(98)80057-6

[93] Santhiago MR, Wilson SE, Smadja D, Chamon W, Krueger RE, Randleman JB. Validation of the percent tissue altered as a risk factor for ectasia after LASIK. Ophthalmology. 2019;**126**(6):908-909. DOI: 10.1016/j.ophtha.2019.01.018

[94] Cohen E, Spierer O. Dry eye post-laser-assisted in situ keratomileusis: Major review and latest updates. Journal of Ophthalmology. 2018;**2018**:4903831. [Accessed: January 28, 2018]. DOI: 10.1155/2018/4903831

[95] Albietz JM, Lenton LM, McLennan SG. Chronic dry eye and regression after laser in situ keratomileusis for myopia. Journal of Cataract and Refractive Surgery. 2004;**30**(3):675-684. DOI: 10.1016/j.jcrs.2003.07.003

[96] Albietz JM, Lenton LM. Management of the ocular surface and tear film before, during, and after laser in situ keratomileusis. Journal of Refractive Surgery. 2004;**20**(1):62-71. DOI: 10.3928/1081-597X-20040101-11

[97] Raoof D, Pineda R. Dry eye after laser in-situ keratomileusis. Seminars in Ophthalmology. 2014;**29**(5-6):358-362. DOI: 10.3109/08820538.2014.962663

[98] Shtein RM. Post-LASIK dry eye. Expert Review of Ophthalmology. 2011;**6**(5):575-582. DOI: 10.1586/eop.11.56

[99] Darwish T, Brahma A, O'Donnell C, Efron N. Subbasal nerve fiber regeneration after LASIK and LASEK assessed by noncontact esthesiometry and in vivo confocal microscopy: Prospective study. Journal of Cataract and Refractive Surgery. 2007;**33**(9):1515-1521. DOI: 10.1016/j.jcrs.2007.05.023

[100] Salib GM, McDonald MB, Smolek M. Safety and efficacy of cyclosporine 0.05% drops versus unpreserved artificial tears in dry-eye patients having laser in situ keratomileusis. Journal of Cataract and Refractive Surgery. 2006;**32**(5):772-778. DOI: 10.1016/j.jcrs.2005.10.034

[101] Myung D, Schallhorn S, Manche EE. Pupil size and LASIK: A review. Journal of Refractive Surgery. 2013;**29**(11):734-741. DOI: 10.3928/1081597X-20131021-02

[102] Miraftab M, Fotouhi A, Hashemi H, Jafari F, Shahnazi A, Asgari S. A modified risk assessment scoring system for post laser in situ keratomileusis ectasia in topographically normal patients. Journal of Ophthalmic and Vision Research. 2014;**9**(4):434-438. DOI: 10.4103/2008-322X.150806

[103] Pop M, Payette Y. Risk factors for night vision complaints after LASIK for myopia. Ophthalmology. 2004;**111**(1):3-10. DOI: 10.1016/j.ophtha.2003.09.022

[104] Schallhorn SC, Tanzer DJ, Kaupp SE, Brown M, Malady SE. Comparison of night driving performance after wavefront-guided and conventional LASIK for moderate myopia. Ophthalmology. 2009;**116**(4):702-709. DOI: 10.1016/j.ophtha.2008.12.038

Section 4

Intraocular Refractive Surgery - Special Cases

Chapter 5

Surgical Correction of Ametropia with AddOn™ Intraocular Lens in Post-Penetrating Keratoplasty Pseudophakia

Iva Dekaris, Ivan Gabrić and Doria Gabrić

Abstract

Cataract surgery is the most common surgery in ophthalmology. The aim of cataract surgery is to restore vision in eyes in which the natural lens became opacified mostly due to the aging of the lens, or the presence of other ocular diseases, which promote earlier cataract formation. During cataract surgery, artificial intraocular lens (IOL) is implanted into the lens capsule and the value of the IOL is planned before surgery based on the preoperative IOL calculation. However, in the significant number of patients, cataract surgery may end up with a postoperative refractive error in which case patients have to wear glasses to reach the full vision for both distance and near correction (if monofocal IOL is used during cataract surgery!). Modern cataract surgery becomes more and more a refractive procedure as well, especially when multifocal and/or toric IOLs are implanted. However, in some specific cases where such IOLs are not applicable, high postoperative refractive error after cataract surgery can significantly influence the quality of the obtained vision. One such example is cataract surgery after penetrating keratoplasty. In this chapter, results of a novel approach of post-PK ametropia correction, namely implantation of sulcus placed AddOn IOLs (also called a piggyback lens) will be presented.

Keywords: AddOn IOL, penetrating keratoplasty, ametropia, refractive error, piggyback lens

1. Introduction

In patients who have had penetrating keratoplasty (PK) cataract surgery cannot end up in emmetropia due to the fact that they all have significant postoperative astigmatism due to the presence of corneal graft. In eyes without corneal graft, which have significant astigmatism, the problem can be solved with the implantation of monofocal toric IOL, which can correct higher amounts of astigmatism. However, in patients with corneal graft, it is questionable whether to use monofocal toric IOL since we never know whether corneal graft will survive throughout patient life, or the graft will need to be changed later during patients' life. If the graft needs to be changed and we have already implanted toric IOL during cataract surgery adjusted to the refractive error of the first corneal graft, the patient would have non-appropriate toric IOL in the eye. Thus, for patients with corneal graft, which develop cataract, we need a "reversible" correction of pre-existing astigmatism and, for that purpose, piggyback or AddOn IOLs are almost ideal option. Namely, AddOn IOLs can be easily and safely implanted in the ciliary sulcus over the already existing "in-the-bag" monofocal IOL, and if needed, they can be safely removed later on [1]. Thus, our method of choice for ametropia correction in post-PK patients who cannot wear contact lenses or spectacles to solve their ametropia is the implantation of AddOn IOL in the ciliary sulcus. This type of lens is used in eyes that already have had cataract surgery with implantation of conventional monofocal IOL in-the-bag. In this chapter, all the main aspects of add-on IOL usage in such cases are clarified.

2. Characteristics of 1stQ AddOn lens

The 1stQ AddOn is a single-piece hydrophilic monofocal IOL for implantation into the ciliary sulcus in addition to a primary IOL in the patient's pseudophakic eye (Medicontur). This lens is implanted into the ciliary sulcus in addition to the IOL in the capsular bag and it is compatible with common capsular bag IOL, irrespective of design or material (**Figure 1**). Due to the lens convex-concave design, a space between AddOn IOL and posterior chamber IOL is approximately 0.5 mm, so there is no touch between the optics of the two implanted lenses. 1stQ AddOn lens is appropriate for the correction of both spherical refractive errors and astigmatism [1, 2]. The AddOn power calculation is typically made with the help of 1stQ AddOn®Calculator for the calculation of sulcus-fixated AddOn® IOLs. However, due to the fact that the amount of astigmatism is unusually "high" after PK, the calculation of the lens power for our specific cases was made by the manufacturer (Medicontur) and not by the operating surgeon. In post-penetrating keratoplasty cases, it was always implanted in the pseudophakic eye, although this type of lens can also be implanted in a single procedure namely together with the extraction of cataract (for example if the lens is used to correct presbyopia!). This type of IOL is very safe to implant into the sulcus due to the four important features: the lens has four flexible haptics, very good rotational stability due to its non-torque design, it is of convex-concave optic design enabling no IOL touch of adjacent eye structures, and it has square design making it safe regarding

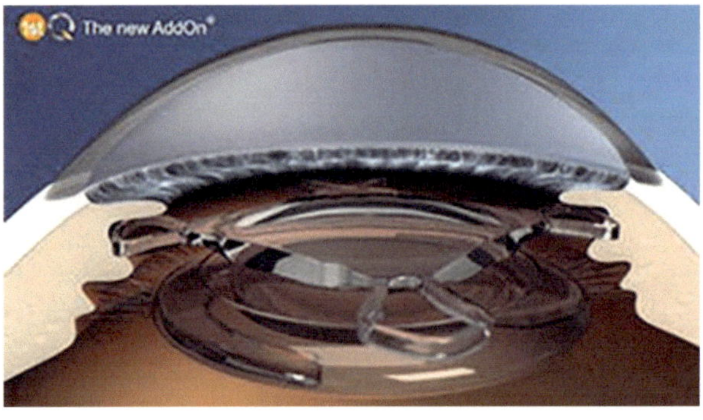

Figure 1.
Position of 1stQ Addon lens in the ciliary sulcus (www.medicontur.com).

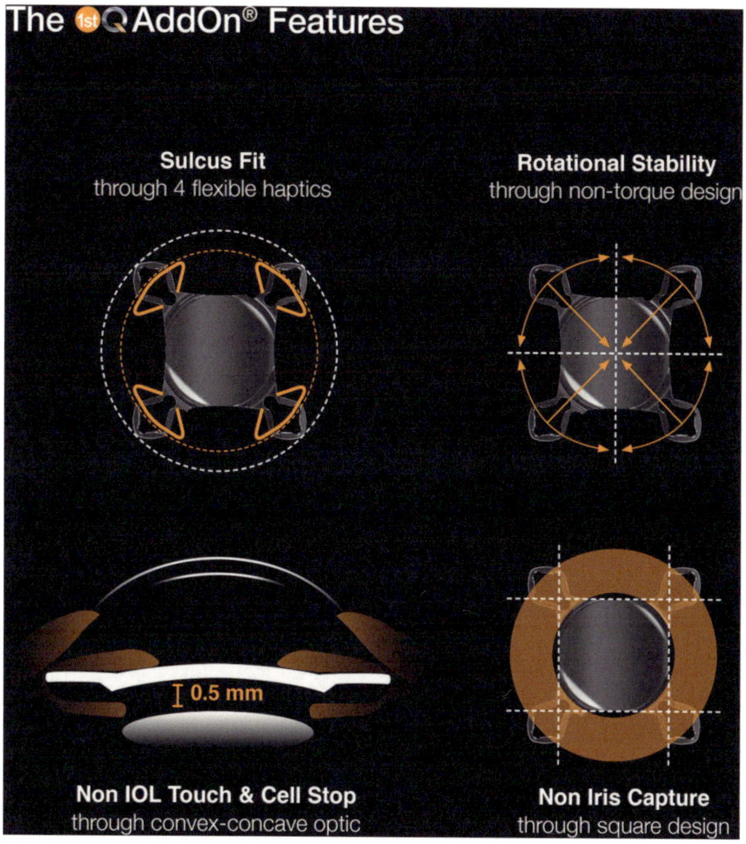

Figure 2.
main characteristics of 1stQ Addon lens (www.medicontur.com).

touch of the iris ("no iris capture" design) (**Figure 2**). The lens can be positioned safely irrespective of the size and shape of the ciliary sulcus [1–3].

3. Surgical procedure

Implantation of AddOn IOL was always performed under topical anesthesia. The anterior chamber was filled with dispersive (on the corneal endothelium!) and cohesive viscoelastic after side-ports were formed. The incision size was 2.4–2.7 mm. The lens was loaded into the lens injector with viscoelastic and the tip of the injector was placed intracamerally prior to the insertion of AddOn IOL. The lens was injected very slowly in order to allow the leading haptic to unfold in a controlled manner and then the haptic was guided under the iris (**Figure 3**) [1]. During the injection procedure, care was taken not to push against the primary lens to maintain zonular stability. Due to its design, toric versions of the lens are easier to rotate into position without all four haptics positioned in the sulcus; thus, the lens was rotated into its desired position before placement of the other two haptics behind the iris. The lens could be rotated in either direction. Once the desired position of the toric lens was obtained, the other 2 haptics were also gently placed into the sulcus behind the iris, and a careful check-up was made to be sure that all four haptics are positioned behind the iris. It was very important to check that all

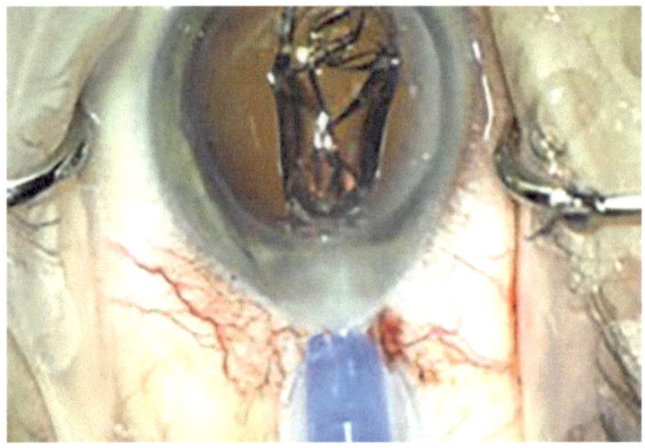

Figure 3.
Implantation of a 1stQ Addon lens with the Medicel Accuject 2.1 injector (www.medicontur.com).

four haptics are positioned behind the iris before removing the viscoelastic, particularly in our patients with corneal transplants, as it may be difficult to see the haptics behind the corneal scar. Some pearls for insertion include the use of the microscope with an integrated OCT image; thus, the surgeon can visualize the sulcus and position of the AddOn lens in the sulcus intraoperatively with the highest precision. It is also important to have good pupil dilation, and careful manipulation with the lens since in post-PK eyes special attention is needed not to destroy any endothelial cells during lens implantation. The advantage of post-PK eyes was that all the eyes had a very deep anterior chamber with enough space for manipulation with the lens.

4. Ametropia correction in post-PK eyes

We have used AddOn IOL in post-PK eyes with a significant refractive error that could not be corrected by contact lens or spectacle wear. All of our post-PK eyes in which AddOn lens was implanted gained significant improvement in their non-corrected distance visual acuity and the satisfaction rate was extremely high. Implantation of the AddOn lens had no influence on near visual acuity and low-contrast

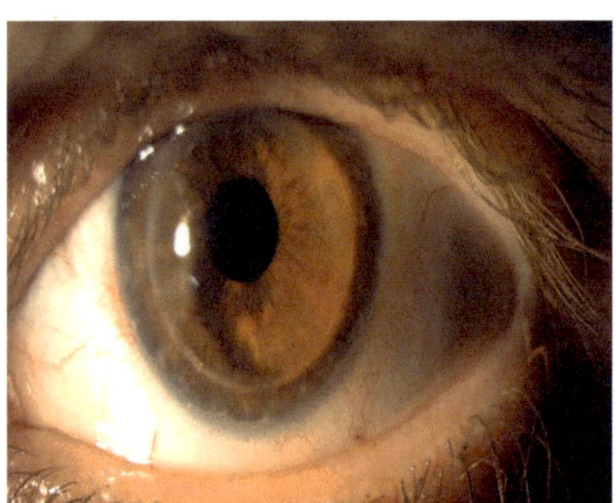

Figure 4.
Slit-lamp image of the eye in which penetrating keratoplasty and cataract surgery with posterior chamber IOL implantation was done.

acuity. A typical example of a post-PK eye in which cataract was already removed and posterior chamber IOL implanted in the capsular bag is shown in **Figure 4**, together with its corneal topography (measured by Pentacam) showing significant post-PK astigmatism (**Figure 5**). For each post-PK eye an individual Addon lens is ordered and produced according to patients' individual measurements (**Figure 6a** and **b**). Lens implantation is made according to the previously described surgical procedure. The position of the lens after the surgery can be precisely checked postoperatively on the OCT scan of the anterior eye chamber to control for a proper distance between AddOn lens and PCIOL (**Figure 7**). The results of the significant increase in visual acuity in our first 3 post-PK eyes implanted with Addon IOL are represented in **Figure 8**. A dramatic increase in visual acuity from preoperative non-corrected (VA sc preop) is represented.

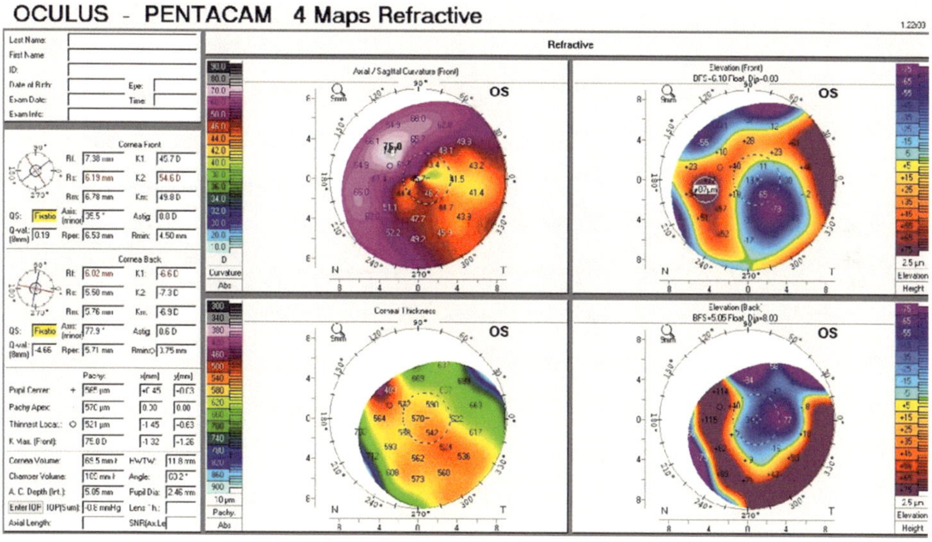

Figure 5.
Corneal topography of a post-PK pseudophakic eye showing significant astigmatism which can be corrected with Addon lens implantation.

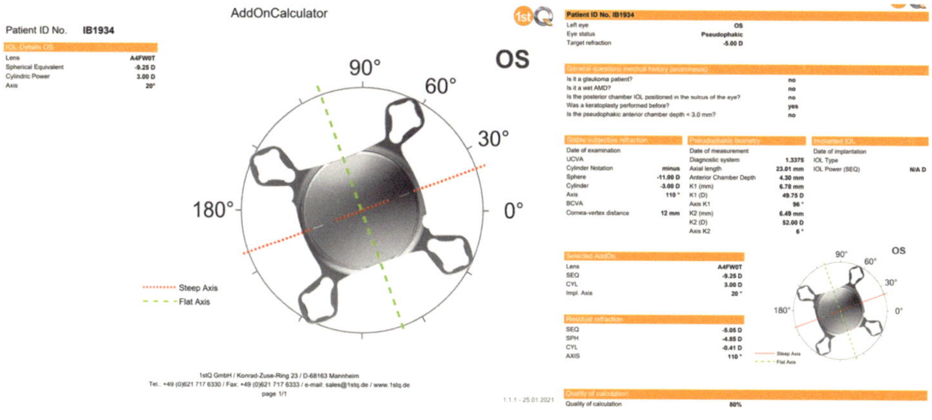

Figure 6.
(a, b) Individual patient data and the outcome measurements for the individually designed Addon provided by manufacturer.

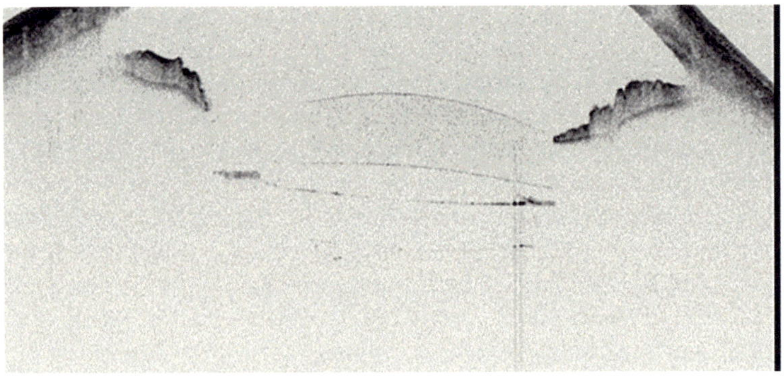

Figure 7.
OCT image showing position of AddOn IOL and the already existing PCIOL with adequate distance between the two lenses.

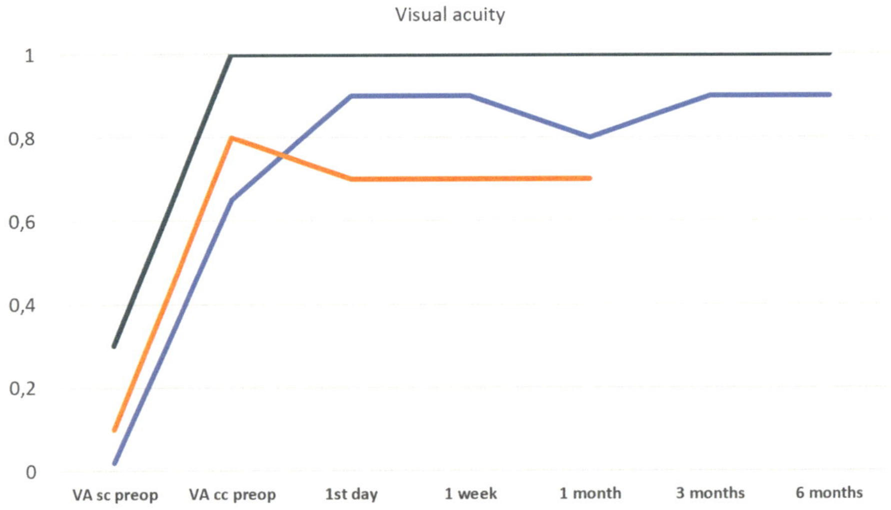

Figure 8.
Change in visual acuity after AddOn lens implantation in 3 representative post-PK cases.

The preoperative best-corrected (VA cc preop) is a vision tested by an eye doctor in the office; however, none of the patients could in fact wear such a correction in a real-life situation since their eyes did not support correction with either contact lens or spectacles. Therefore, their vision of 5–15% prior to AddOn lens implantation increased to 80–100% vision after AddOn lens implantation. As expected, with such a dramatic change in vision all patients were extremely satisfied with the outcome of the surgery. Those results are comparable with other publications [3–5].

Since patients with AddOn IOL in fact have two lenses in the eye; and despite the fact that AddOn IOL is very gentle and thin, we checked whether intraocular pressure (IOP) is increased by implantation of such lens and according to our results AddOn lens did not change values of IOP in 6 postoperative months of patients' follow-up (**Figure 9**). A typical sample of corneal endothelial cell count pre- and post- Addon IOL implantation is shown in **Figure 10**. Due to the very deep anterior chamber in all post-PK eyes, the surgery of Addon IOL implantation did not influence the regularity and count of corneal endothelial cells.

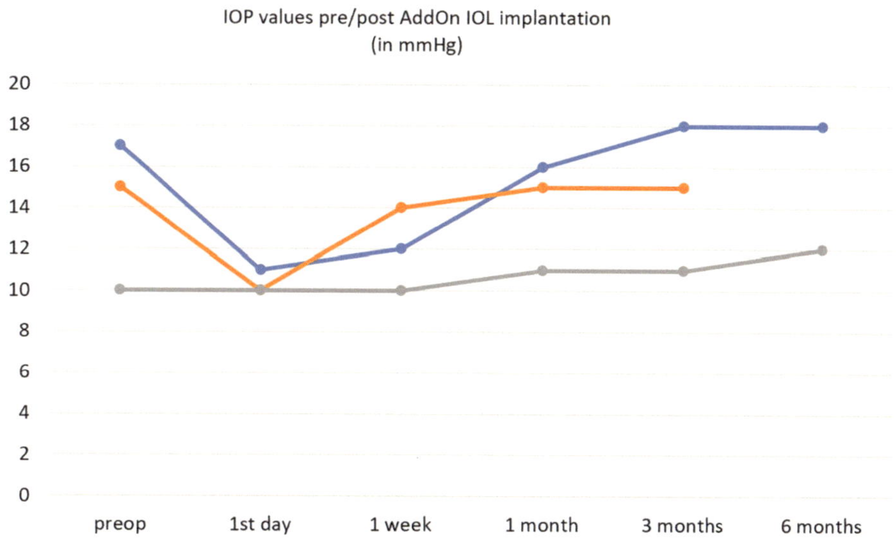

Figure 9.
Intraoperative pressure (IOP) values before and after Addon IOL implantation.

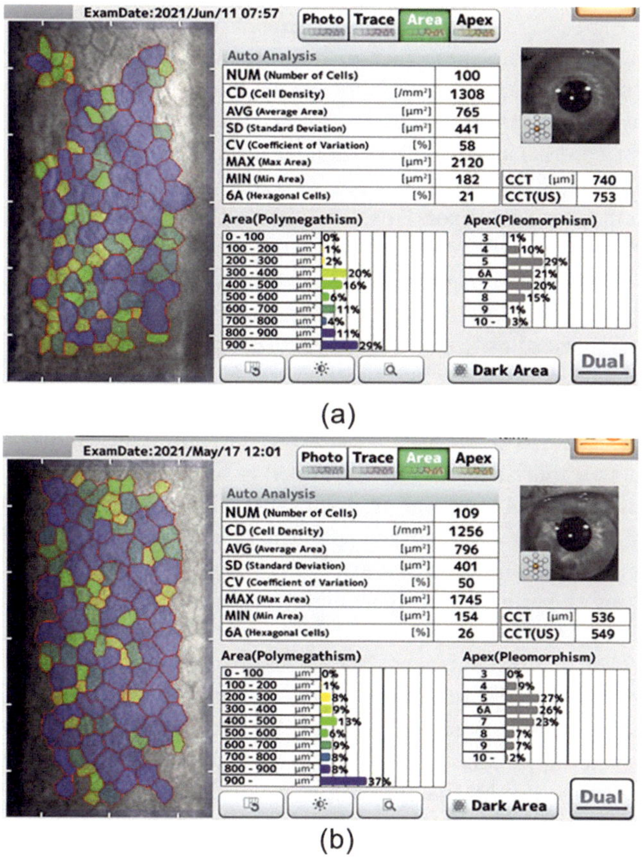

Figure 10.
Endothelial cell density count pre- (10a) and post- (10b) AddOn IOL implantation.

5. Discussion

Penetrating keratoplasty can be a life-changing procedure for those patients who suffer from significant vision loss due to a corneal disease involving all corneal layers. Despite the fact that the success of this procedure may be limited by some postoperative complications like graft rejection, postoperative rise in intraocular pressure, or cataract formation, most of the patients with a clear corneal graft are extremely satisfied with their improvement of vision. In some cases, however, despite of the fact that the corneal graft is perfectly clear and there have been no postoperative complications jeopardizing the quality of the grafted tissue, we may end up with very unsatisfied patients with very low uncorrected visual acuity equal to or even worse as compared to preoperative vision. This happens in eyes with a corneal graft having very high postoperative astigmatism which cannot be corrected with a contact lens. Most often such cases develop after suturing of the graft with interrupted sutures or with the unexpected change in astigmatism after suture removal. We must bear in mind that the astigmatism is not only the result of the suture placement, but also a result of the type of healing process in each particular eye, so it may be that the patient has good vision and a low amount of astigmatism for a several months after surgery and then, unfortunately, develops a high astigmatism. Similarly, at the time of suture removal, we cannot judge the amount of astigmatism which will remain after suture removal. Recently new types of contact lens such as scleral lens has been developed to help in cases with very high astigmatism, but still, some patients remain who are not able to wear such lenses and who are in fact without any solution to improve their vision after PK. With the invention of AddOn lenses, which were primarily designed to correct refractive errors after more often performed surgeries like cataract surgery, corneal surgeons could also start to use such lenses for their post-PK patients. AddOn lenses are produced in a personalized manner as previously said, and according to individual patient refractive error. However, due to the high amount of astigmatism in some of post-PK cases it may happen that the manufacturer does not have an option of producing a lens for full astigmatism correction. We have also had such patients which were consequently "under-corrected" regarding their astigmatism. However, even if the full amount of astigmatism is not corrected with the AddOn lens, those patients still gained significantly better postoperative vision and were perfectly happy with obtained vision. Moreover, since in many of post-PK cases we do not have a regular type of astigmatism, we were worried that the outcome may not be as good as if the regular astigmatism is corrected. This is easily visible in **Figure 5**, where the irregularity of the post-PK astigmatism is clearly visible. However, clinically, despite the irregularity of post-PK astigmatism the visual outcome was better than expected and the patient satisfaction rate was high. Therefore, the AddOn lenses are the best and truly speaking the only currently available option for post-PK cases with high astigmatism, being of regular type (which is in fact rarely seen) or of the irregular type. The drawback of AddOn lenses that we have noticed was that the lens is not produced for extremely high amounts of astigmatism (>10 dioptres) and such high astigmatism may be seen in post-PK patients. Thus, the production of AddOn lens able to correct even higher amounts of astigmatism would be an improvement in 1stQAddOn lens portfolio. All the operated eyes, as mentioned before, were pseudophakic. We do know from the literature that refractive errors in pseudophakic eyes can sometimes be corrected with the replacement of the existing IOL. However, in post-PK cases, this is not an option since we would need to replace the IOL with toric IOL. However, in post-PK cases, the graft may be replaced in the future and then the toric IOL in the eye would be certainly not appropriate since astigmatism after repeated PK cannot be the same. Since AddOn lenses are not in use for a longer period of time for post-PK cases we still cannot comment on the performance of those lenses in a longer follow-up and this remains to be studied in the future. Namely, a follow-up of 6 months (which we have presented in this chapter) on the effect of AddOn lenses on postoperative IOP and on the state of endothelial cells should be studied in a long run as well.

6. Conclusion

Implantation of AddOn IOL in pseudophakic eyes with post-PK refractive error is safe and easy procedure to significantly improve visual acuity in post-PK cases unable to wear contact lenses or spectacles (at least for the shorter follow-up). Also, there was no adverse effect or IOP rise, and one of the main advantages is its reversibility in case of the next transplantation.

Author details

Iva Dekaris*, Ivan Gabrić and Doria Gabrić
University Eye Hospital Svjetlost, Zagreb, Croatia

*Address all correspondence to: iva.dekaris@svjetlost.hr

References

[1] Instruction for use 1stQ addon IOL ... – implantecinsumos.com [Internet]. 1stQ AddOn® IOL. 1stQ GmbH; 2015. Available from: https://implantecinsumos.com/wp-content/uploads/2019/10/ifu_1stq_iol_addon_en_20150908.pdf. [Accessed: March 19, 2022]

[2] Themes UFO. Addon® intraocular lenses [Internet]. Ento Key. 2017. Available from: https://entokey.com/addon-intraocular-lenses/. [Accessed: March 19, 2022]

[3] Gundersen KG, Potvin R. Refractive and visual outcomes after implantation of a secondary toric sulcus intraocular lenses. Clinical Ophthalmology. 2020;**14**:1337-1342

[4] Hassenstein A, Niemeck F, Giannakakis K, Klemm M. Torische addon-Intraokularlinsen zur Korrektur Hoher Astigmatismen nach Pseudophaker Keratoplastik. Der Ophthalmologe. 2016;**114**(6):549-555

[5] Srinivasan S, Ting DS, Lyall DA. Implantation of a customized Toric intraocular lens for correction of post-keratoplasty astigmatism. Eye. 2013;**27**(4):531-537

Chapter 6

Refractive Lensectomy and Microinvasive Glaucoma Surgery (MIGS): An Initial Approach in Glaucoma Patients over 50 Years of Age

Daniel Laroche and Kara Rickford

Abstract

Glaucoma is a common cause of blindness worldwide, affecting patients at an average age of 57 years old. This is a disease of ocular anatomy commonly caused by a blockage of trabecular meshwork leading to an increase in intraocular pressure and glaucomatous optic neuropathy. The lens enlarges in width with age, often contributing to this, with obstruction of the angle due to pupillary block in angle-closure glaucoma. In open-angle glaucoma, there is often increased pigment liberation and obstruction of the trabecular meshwork due to increased iridolenticular and zonular contact. Recent studies looking at cataract extraction, refractive lensectomy, and the Hydrus stent have demonstrated adequate safety and efficacy for the treatment of glaucoma. We review the latest glaucoma treatment algorithm and results with early cataract surgery/refractive lensectomy and microinvasive glaucoma surgery to be considered as initial treatment for patients with glaucoma over 50 years of age.

Keywords: glaucoma, refractive lensectomy, microinvasive glaucoma surgery, MIGS

1. Introduction

Glaucoma is a progressive and chronic optic neuropathy characterized by degeneration of the inner layers of the retina, specifically the retinal ganglion cells [1, 2]. As these cells and their axons degenerate with increasing age, the risk of vision loss increases. As a leading cause of blindness worldwide, glaucoma cases are predicted to grow with the increasing aging population by more than double between 2010 and 2050 in the United States [3].

Glaucoma most commonly occurs in people over the age of 40 and rises in prevalence as people age. Natural aging leads to altered age-associated ocular tissue, such as the extracellular matrix. In glaucoma, extensive extracellular matrix remodeling takes place in the trabecular meshwork and the optic nerve leading to tissue stiffening and fibrosis that can cause an increase in intraocular pressure [2, 4]. Additionally, with age, the lens enlarges in width and volume causing greater iridolenticular and iridozonular contact during accommodation [5, 6]. This increased contact leads to pigment liberation that can obstruct the trabecular meshwork and lead to the narrowing of anterior angle structures [5]. Although the outcomes of this ocular pathology can be severe, population-level surveys have demonstrated that many people with glaucoma are unaware that they have it due to its asymptomatic progressive manner [7, 8]. In addition to age, the prevalence of glaucoma cases is higher in Black Americans and individuals of African descent are at higher risk than other races for developing primary open-angle glaucoma [3, 9].

While early treatment of glaucoma has shown to be efficacious, no treatment yet exists for restoring loss of vision of glaucomatous optic neuropathy, therefore emphasizing the importance of early intervention and prevention of vision loss. The standard treatment for glaucoma is trabeculectomy, which is an ocular surgical technique performed to create a new pathway for fluid within the eye to be drained subconjunctivally with associated risks and complications [10]. Recent studies looking at cataract extraction/refractive lensectomy and the Hydrus stent have demonstrated strong safety and efficacy as a novel earlier treatment of glaucoma [11, 12]. This chapter will explore the current literature to report the use of refractive lensectomy in combination with microinvasive glaucoma surgery (MIGS) as an earlier and initial treatment for glaucoma thereby reducing the need for trabeculectomy.

2. Current treatment options for glaucoma

The two most common types of age-related primary glaucomas include open-angle glaucoma and angle-closure glaucoma. Primary open-angle glaucoma (POAG) is the most common type in the United States, affecting nine out of 10 people with glaucoma [13]. The mean normal intraocular pressure (IOP) is 15 mmHg and individuals with untreated glaucoma present with a mean normal IOP of 18 mmHg [14]. Both of these groups of patients often have age-related enlarged lenses contributing to the obstruction of the trabecular meshwork mechanically or with increased particulate trabecular meshwork pigment. According to the American Academy of Ophthalmology, the standard goal to treat POAG is to lower IOP by 25% [15, 16]. We revisit this in this chapter.

2.1 Topical glaucoma medications

While increasing evidence supports the use of Selective Laser Therapy (SLT) as the initial treatment for POAG, topical medications are of the most utilized treatments for glaucoma [17]. Topical eye drops within the drug classes of beta-blockers, diuretics, cholinergic agonists, alpha agonists, rho-kinase inhibitors, and prostaglandin analogs have been used to lower IOP [18]. Of these, prostaglandin analogs have shown greater efficacy than beta-blockers in reducing IOP with fewer systemic side effects [19, 20]. If monotherapy is not effective, additional topical drugs have been added in conjunction to reduce IOP. Although these pharmacologic agents have demonstrated success in reducing the rate of visual field loss, studies examining the results from the Early Manifest Glaucoma trial have shown disease progression despite reduced IOP [21]. Additionally, topical medications for glaucoma require reliable patient adherence to reap the benefits [22]. Previous studies have recognized decreased patient adherence with an increasing number of prescribed topicals to treat glaucoma [23]. Other studies have shown that medication adherence in glaucoma patients is affected by disease severity, demonstrating that those with the most severe disease had higher levels of adherence [22]. These findings challenge the vast benefits of treating glaucoma early with topical medications. If patients with mild glaucoma are less likely to adhere to topical medication treatment, the susceptibility to disease progression increases. Topical medications have also been shown to increase the risk of cataract formation [24]. Despite the initial lowering of intraocular pressure, patients with this side effect can have worsening enlargement of the lens with increased pigment liberation from iridolenticular rubbing or narrowing of the angle, potentially worsening trabecular meshwork outflow.

A long-term history of topical glaucoma medication use and high preoperative glaucoma drug scores have been recognized as a risk factors for surgical failure of trabeculotomy [25–28]. In a recent study conducted by Okuda et al., researchers examined the perioperative factors that affected the surgical success of ab-interno microhook trabeculotomy. The findings revealed that patients taking anti-glaucoma eye drop medications for more than 4.5 years had a lower success rate of cataract surgery and microinvasive trabeculectomy [25]. These findings may be attributed to the substances found within glaucoma eye drops, such as benzalkonium chloride (BAK), that can cause prolonged inflammation and damage to the drainage of the aqueous humor through Schlemm's canal. Preceding studies have suggested that the mechanism by which BAK prolongs inflammation is through an increase in the number of tissue regulators, such as conjunctival macrophages, fibroblasts, and lymphocytes, and a decrease in the number of conjunctival goblet cells that lubricate the ocular surface [26–29]. Other studies have found that BAK may affect aqueous outflow by increasing oxidative stress in the cells of the trabecular meshwork and endothelium, leading to apoptosis and an eventual increase in IOP [30, 31]. Therefore, the effects of chronic inflammation caused by prolonged glaucoma medication use can lead to remodeling of the aqueous humor outflow pathway, and eventually antagonize the opening of the trabecular meshwork during a trabeculectomy or distal outflow after a Schlemm's canal procedure [25].

Additional reports have suggested that the outflow pathway may undergo disuse atrophy with extended glaucoma medication use. The most commonly used topical eye drops for glaucoma, with the exception of rho-kinase inhibitors, relieve ocular pressure by reducing the production of aqueous humor and promoting its drainage through the uveoscleral pathway [32]. Consequently, prolonged use of these medications may lead to disuse atrophy of the pathway of Schlemm's canal, which should typically function to collect the aqueous humor from the anterior chamber of the eye. As such, this can lead to complications with filtration surgery, as demonstrated by Johnson and Matsumoto [33], who recognized a decrease in the size of Schlemm's canal following filtration surgery. Their findings demonstrated that following successful surgery, the aqueous outflow enters the filtration bleb and bypasses the trabecular meshwork and canal resulting in under perfusion and eventual atrophy of these structures [33]. The prolonged use of topical glaucoma medications decreases the success rate of filtration surgeries due to the remodeling, inflammation, and eventual dysfunction of these pathways. It is, therefore, imperative that glaucoma medications be prescribed responsibly, particularly with long-term use, and other treatment options are considered to avoid potential issues with poor adherence or overuse.

2.2 Laser therapies

Laser therapies are used to treat glaucoma by targeting thermal energy toward the trabecular meshwork to open the space in adjacent structures and improve outflow [34]. This therapy was first used in response to high IOPs that were not reduced in response to medical management. Today, laser therapies are used earlier in disease progression without waiting for maximal medical management [35]. The most common form of laser surgery used is Selective Laser trabeculoplasty (SLT), which is used as both a primary and adjunct therapy [36]. This treatment option has been shown to be cost-effective in comparison to medical therapy [37, 38] and shows similar outcomes in reducing IOP [39]. However, SLT has been shown to have a low success rate in treating advanced glaucoma, in particular, following the use of multiple glaucoma medications. Furthermore, the reported predictors of success in SLT treatment have shown conflicting findings [40, 41].

There are several possible reasons for conflicting results with SLT treatment. First, higher success rates using SLT have been demonstrated in patients with the earlier disease and higher baseline IOP (above 22 mmHg) [36, 42, 43]. Furthermore, SLT therapy may have higher rates of failure when treating patients with lower baseline IOPs and more advanced disease [40], therefore, inferring that this therapeutic option may be less efficacious in some patients. Additionally, many confounding variables may affect the success rate of laser therapy today that were not present many years ago. As noted by Song et al., many individuals undergoing glaucoma treatment may be taking a newer class of drugs, such as prostaglandin agonists, α-2 adrenergic agonists, or topical carbonic anhydrase inhibitors, that may contribute to the higher failure rate of SLT therapy today in comparison to 20–30 years ago [40, 44–46]. In addition, findings from the Laser in Glaucoma and Ocular Hypertension (LiGHT) trial have revealed that despite successful SLT at 6 years, 19.7% of patients still progressed with their glaucoma compared to 26.8% with eyedrop therapy (SLT LiGHT trial 6-year data presented at American Glaucoma Society March 2021, Nashville, Tennessee).

Other laser therapies that are currently being studied include titanium-sapphire laser trabeculoplasty, pattern scanning trabeculoplasty, and cyclophotocoagulation [35]. Of these, cyclophotocoagulation is increasingly being used by glaucoma surgeons in combination with other therapies [47, 48]. Although micropulse transscleral cyclophotocoagulation (MPTCP) has been used to reduce IOP [49, 50], studies have shown low success rates with repeated treatments [50–52]. A retrospective case series conducted at the National University of Singapore found low rates of success in lowering IOP despite multiple attempts at MPTCP [52]. Additionally, the IOP-lowering effects of repeated MPTCP were short-lasting with a median time of 4.6 months [52]. The safety and efficacy of this treatment are dependent on the duration and power settings of the laser, which has differed between studies [51, 52]. In comparison to continuous-wave transscleral cyclophotocoagulation and endocyclophotocoagulation, MPTCP has been shown to have a better safety profile [53, 54]. Complications associated with MPTCP may be due to repeated treatments of energy on the targeted pigmented tissues, particularly if the duration between consecutive treatments is short [52, 53, 55]. While the MPTCP is an overall safe option with only mild risks of ocular complications, the short longevity span of reduced IOP suggests other treatment options can have better long-term efficacy for glaucoma patients.

2.3 Trabeculectomy

The gold standard for treating glaucoma has traditionally been trabeculectomy for filtration surgery. While topical eyedrop and or SLT can slow progression, surgery may be required for cases that do not respond to these treatments or are more severe.

The findings in the Collaborative Initial Glaucoma Treatment study [56] and the Advanced Glaucoma Intervention Study [57] concluded that glaucomatous visual field deterioration could be reduced with trabeculectomy. Despite its popularity, many risk factors including higher preoperative IOP, postoperative inflammation, younger age, and diabetes were associated with a higher rate of trabeculectomy failure [57]. The risk of requiring cataract surgery following trabeculectomy surgery is reported between 20% and 52% postoperatively. Furthermore, the Collaborative Normal-Tension Glaucoma Study [58] and the Collaborative Initial Glaucoma Treatment Study [59] have demonstrated an increased incidence of cataracts in individuals who had undergone filtration surgery. Other side effects of trabeculectomy, as summarized by Chou et al., include blebitis, blebitis-associated endophthalmitis, diplopia, tube erosions, damage to the corneal endothelium, and hypotony [60]. Although trabeculectomy is effective in reducing IOP in patients with open-angle glaucoma, the higher incidence of short- and long-term complications offer the possibility of exploring further treatments for glaucoma. Due to its efficacy in treating normal-tension glaucoma (NTG) and achieving low intraocular pressure in patients with advanced glaucoma, the use of trabeculectomy is important and will likely persist. Trabeculectomy also offers better IOP lowering compared to the Xen 45 Gel stent [61].

2.4 Drainage implants for glaucoma

Glaucoma drainage implants (GDI) were once more commonly used to treat refractory glaucoma. These work by using a tube to divert the aqueous humor from the anterior chamber of the eye. The Tube versus Trabeculectomy (TVT) Study [62] demonstrated the shift in practice patterns to the use of GDI. The study found that patients who had a previous trabeculectomy and/or cataract extraction with uncontrolled glaucoma (>18 mmHg) had better success with tube shunt surgery in a 5-year follow-up than those who underwent trabeculectomy. The findings revealed a 29.8% probability of failure in the group receiving the tube shunt, compared to the 46.9% probability of failure in the group with trabeculectomy [62]. The failure rate for trabeculectomy resembled those shown in previous studies [63–65], while the failure rate of the tube shunt was lower than previously reported [66, 67]. While most GDIs have a similar design, the most commonly used are the Ahmed valve (New World Medical, Inc., Rancho Cucamonga, CA) and the Baerveldt implant (Abbott Medical Optics, Inc., Santa Ana, CA) and have not shown differences in superiority [68]. Drainage tube implants continue to be a very important treatment for glaucoma patients. Since these devices are large and use a substantial amount of conjunctival space, they can cause cataract formation and corneal decompensation. Glaucoma tube shunts are usually performed in conjunction with or preferably after cataract surgery has been performed. In this procedure, placing the tube in the ciliary sulcus, reduces the risk of corneal decompensation [69]. Glaucoma tube shunt surgery has also been reported combined with goniotomy and retrobulbar tube placement [70].

3. Refractive lensectomy and intraocular lens placement

Refractive lensectomy, also referred to as refractive lens exchange or clear lens extraction, is similar to cataract surgery as both procedures involve the removal of the natural lens of the eye and replacing it with a synthetic lens. Individuals with primary angle-closure diseases have a shallow anterior chamber due to a thicker lens in the anterior position [71]. Refractive lensectomy is a surgical procedure that can remove the lens to relieve crowding of the angle and deepen the anterior chamber, as shown in the literature [72, 73]. The EAGLE Study was a prospective multicenter clinical study that found that in patients with angle-closure glaucoma, those who underwent a refractive lensectomy (clear lens extraction with intraocular lens) presented with a lower IOP and less medication than patients in the iridotomy group [74]. This surgical procedure also plays a role as a solution to a refractive error in hyperopia, particularly in patients with narrow angles. Glaucoma patients with high degrees of myopia and hyperopia can also benefit from an improved vision from refractive lensectomy and associated intraocular pressure lowering. We further review the use of refractive surgery in patients with myopia and hyperopia.

3.1 Refractive lensectomy in myopia

Myopia, commonly referred to as nearsightedness, is a refractive error that occurs when the eye does not focus light properly on the retina. When mild, this is referred to as mild myopia and when severe, this is referred to as high myopia, which typically stabilizes between the ages of 20–30 years old [75]. Refractive lensectomy has been used to correct high myopia, particularly among those who are approaching or currently have presbyopia [76]. The procedure is performed by skilled experienced surgeons using modern phacoemulsification techniques and causes less disturbances to the homeostasis of the eye by using small incision sizes, improved stability in the anterior chamber, and foldable intraocular lenses [76, 77].

Many studies and reviews have assessed the results and risks of lens refractive procedures, as summarized by Alio et al. [76]. Jean Arne compared phakic intraocular lens (IOL) implantation with clear lens extraction (CLE) in 39 patients aged 30–50 years old and found a lower risk for loss of best correct visual acuity (BCVA) in the phakic IOL group at the one-year follow up [78]. In another study comparing refractive lens exchange (RLE) and Collamer lens (Visian) implantation in patients with myopia younger than 45 years old, the results revealed better outcomes in patients who underwent RLE [79]. In this study, patients in the RLE group experienced no serious complications, while those with the Visian implantation demonstrated pigment dispersion, lens opacity, macular hemorrhage, or pupillary block glaucoma [79]. Additional studies examining the efficacy of RLE have demonstrated encouraging results and revealed a rapid and predictable improvement in vision in patients with high myopia as demonstrated by improved corrected distance visual acuity [77, 80–82].

Although the complications associated with this surgery have a low incidence [83], the visual consequences, lest they occur, may present with real sight-threatening risks including endophthalmitis, intraoperative suprachoroidal hemorrhage, and retinal detachment (RD) [77]. RD is a most common vision-threatening complication of RLE and can occur more commonly in eyes with myopia greater than −10.0 D in unoperated eyes and in eyes following cataract extraction with IOL implantation [76, 84]. The hypothesized reasons behind the increased risk for RD include the increased risk for myopic eyes for predisposed retinal lesions, as well as the induction of iatrogenic factors following refractive surgery [84]. To avoid these complications, the state of the vitreous body should be assessed through preoperative funduscopic examination. The following guidelines were provided by Alios et al. [76] for when to avoid RLE in myopic eyes:

- Eyes with advanced peripheral lattice degenerations
- Young eyes with no posterior vitreous detachment
- Lacquer cracks in high myopia or myopic CNV in the fellow eye
- Presbyopia eyes with macular degeneration beginning in the following eye.

Pre- and postoperative consultation with a retinal specialist can be performed to rule out retinal tears or breaks and prophylactically treat any suspicious retinal degeneration. This has also reduced the risk of retinal detachment [85].

3.1.1 Calculating intraocular lens power

Refractive lens exchange (RLE) requires safety, consistency, and effectiveness during surgery and in the postoperative period for a successful refractive outcome. Accordingly, the accuracy of preoperative procedures for intraocular lens (IOL) power calculations is imperative along with the proper choice of surgical procedure. Kaweri et al. [86] noted that individuals undergoing RLE are comparatively younger and should be advised on the potential loss of accommodation if the monofocal lens is implanted and the photic phenomenon if the multifocal lens is implanted. The surgical technique in RLE is similar to that of cataract surgery and has ideal technical elements that may ensure a successful outcome, as concisely detailed below by Alio et al. [76]

1. Ocular tissues including the corneal endothelium and iris should undergo minimal trauma.
2. Surgically induced or preexisting astigmatisms may be avoided by the surgeon by securing a watertight micro-incision (2.2 mm or less) in a clear cornea about 1.0 mm from the limbus.
3. The posterior chamber IOL should be fixated in the capsular bag, aiming for little to no induction of posterior capsular opacification.

Considerations should be made by the surgeon to address the specific ocular anatomy of the eye, such as those with myopia, extended axial lengths, or hyperopia [76].

3.1.2 Surgical recommendations in high myopia

Eyes with high axial myopia may present with an abnormal depth and stability, requiring the use of a heavy viscoelastic material by surgeons [76]. Many eyes with high myopia have significant astigmatism and may benefit from a temporal approach [86]. Recent advances in clear lens extraction surgery have led to novel approaches in bimanual micro-incisional phacoemulsification. Fine et al. [87] detailed an alternative surgical approach to the traditional coaxial phacoemulsification that involved the removal of the crystalline lens through two 1.2 mm incisions. Using bimanual microincision phacoemulsification, a separate irrigating handpiece can be used for infusion and a sleeveless phacoemulsification needle is used for aspiration and phacoemulsification [87]. This method is conducive to the emulsification and fragmentation of lens material without the generation of significant thermal energy. Additionally, this surgical technique is especially important for patients with a significant risk for retinal detachment following lens extraction, such as those with high myopia [88]. This surgical technique can improve the stability of the chamber, decrease the risk of endophthalmitis, and most importantly reduce the risk of astigmatism induced by surgery [87].

Lens-iris diaphragm retropulsion syndrome may occur during phacoemulsification in highly myopic eyes when the anterior chamber of the eye is deepened, the iris becomes concave, the lens-iris diaphragm is posteriorly displaced, and the pupil dilates in response to the weight of the water column [89]. To avoid this during surgery, the bottle height should be kept low to reduce the infusion limit [89]. Furthermore, an additional instrument may be used to carry out upward tenting of the iris so that the integrity of the ocular structures may be maintained [86]. Capsulorrhexis is used to remove the capsule of the lens of the eye during cataract surgery and should have a 360-degree overlap over the optic in these patients to prevent posterior capsule opacification [90].

The suprascapular approach of phacoemulsification is the preferred, safer method. In this method, the nucleus is prolapsed and emulsified within the anterior chamber [91]. It is recommended that endothelium is coated with viscoelastic prior to phacoemulsification to avoid sudden decompression of the chamber [91]. When compared to the endocapsular technique, the suprascapular approach had an insignificant difference in cell loss, but was more advantageous in cases with zonular weakness and posterior capsular rupture [79]. Accordingly, a successful refractive lens exchange therapy can be achieved with a correctly positioned capsulorrhexis and minimal fluctuations in the anterior chamber [86]. These methods can help maintain the integrity of the ocular structure while minimizing the expenditure of phaco energy.

3.1.3 Selecting the intraocular lens in patients with myopia

In recent years, the growing interest in microincision cataract surgery has led to the increased availability of more flexible IOL. Following refractive lensectomy, a foldable low power lens may be inserted to prevent the development of posterior capsular opacification and the frontward movement of the vitreous [92]. Upon evaluation of the benefits and risk of phacoemulsification to correct high myopia, Fritch found that implantation of an IOL reduced the risk the retinal detachment [93]. The National Outcomes of Cataract Extraction conducted a study that further confirmed these findings and suggested that the probability of retinal detachment following phacoemulsification was less than 1% [94].

Monofocal, toric, and multifocal lenses are used in cataract surgery to replace the natural lens. In refractive lensectomy, a multifocal IOL may be used to achieve contact lens/spectacle independence following surgery and function by distributing light energy into different foci at the expense of contrast sensitivity. When implanting an IOL, it is important to consider the modular transfer function. Trifocal lenses are a subclass of multifocal lenses that have demonstrated excellent near, intermediate, and distant vision but have an inadequate modular transfer in comparison to bifocals [86]. Although in a retrospective study of 787 eyes conducted by Yoon et al. [95], the researchers found that the trifocal diffractive lens demonstrated better intermediate vision than the bifocal diffractive IOL without compromising vision quality.

3.2 Refractive lensectomy in hyperopia

Hyperopia (farsightedness) is a refractive error associated with shallow anterior chambers that are more susceptible to closed-angle glaucoma. Refractive lens surgery corrects high levels of hyperopia through the replacement of the natural lens with an IOL. Hyperopic eyes may benefit from refractive lensectomy due to the increased risk of developing angle-closure glaucoma caused by the small size of the eye and shallow anterior chamber. Several studies have shown satisfactory results in treating hyperopia with refractive lensectomy. Ge et al. compared pseudophakic IOL implant and RLE in the treatment of hyperopia and found that the uncorrected visual acuity was slightly better in the group that underwent RLE and no retinal detachment presented in either group [96]. Fink et al. evaluated refractive lensectomy as a surgical treatment for hyperopia and found refractive lensectomy to be a good alternative to photorefractive keratectomy or laser *in situ* keratomileusis (LASIK) [97]. To follow, Alfonso et al. conducted a prospective study evaluating 41 eyes that underwent RLE following hyperopic LASIK and found that refractive lensectomy following LASIK was safe, effective, and predictable [98]. The safety and efficacy of refractive lensectomy were further confirmed by Preetha et al. [99] and Hoffman et al. [100] through their successful reports of clear lens extraction and bilateral RLE, respectively, in hyperopic eyes.

Similarly, to myopia, ocular pathologies that lead to an increased risk factor for retinal detachment, such as lacquer cracks or lattice degenerations, may be considered contraindications for refractive lensectomy. Additionally, ocular pathologies, such as corneal, diabetic retinopathy, and age-related macular degeneration, can result in poor vision postoperatively, although the risk of postoperative complications in refractive lensectomy is lower than RLE in the treatment of myopia [76, 86, 101].

3.2.1 Surgical recommendations in high hyperopia

Eyes with hyperopia are shorter (axial length < 21 mm) and have an increased risk of macular edema and choroidal effusion during refractive lens exchange [76]. Due to the increased predisposition to closed-angle glaucoma in hyperopic eyes, these individuals are good candidates for RLE, although the complication rate is higher, as demonstrated by Yosar et al. [102]. Hyperopic eyes have an increased risk of developing uveal effusion, iris prolapse, corneal endothelial trauma, cystoid macular edema, and choroidal hemorrhage, making this procedure especially challenging for surgeons [86, 102, 103]. Choroidal hemorrhages may be averted by minimizing fluctuations in the chamber. As with myopia, hyperopic eyes can benefit during surgery from the use of dispersive viscoelastic to the endothelium to prevent damage [86]. Contrastingly, during surgery, a higher bottle height can be used during phacoemulsification to forestall the positive vitreous pressure [86]. A pars plana vitreous tap with an MVR blade and vitrector can deepen the anterior chamber prior to phacoemulsification [104]. Sclerotomy windows can be dissected to reduce the risk of choroidal effusions [105].

More recent reports, including that conducted by Yosar et al., found that cataract surgery in the hyperopic eye was associated with good visual outcomes with a corrected distance visual acuity in 74.6% of study patients, but the complication rate remained higher than that of routine cataract surgery at 25.4% [102]. These findings were further supported by Zhang et al. [106] who found that in patients with malignant glaucoma, using a 23-gauge transconjunctival pars plana vitrectomy combined with lensectomy was a relatively safer manipulation. In comparison to stand-alone lens extraction, the combined surgery was effective by significantly deepening the anterior chamber of the eye (0.507 ± 0.212 mm to 3.080 ± 0.313 mm) and eliminating the blockade of the aqueous in all eyes [106]. Although there was no significant improvement in best-corrected visual acuity at the 21.2 months follow up, the findings also revealed that none of the patients experienced a recurrence of aqueous misdirection, the mean IOP decreased significantly from 43.14 ± 6.53 mmHg to 17.29 ± 1.80 mmHg and the number of postoperative anti-glaucoma medications decreased [106].

Recent studies have contributed to the increasing evidence that lens extraction, in comparison to laser peripheral iridotomy (LPI), may have an advantage. In a retrospective study looking at data from 914 eyes, Ong et al. [107] determined that over 3 years of follow-up, individuals who underwent lens extraction were less likely to experience progression of visual field loss (odds ratio 0.35, 95% confidence interval 0.13–0.91). These patients who received phacoemulsification also required fewer postoperative medications to lower intraocular pressure compared to those with standard care at 12-months. The results of this study also found no additional benefit in combining phacoemulsification with viscogonioplasty, trabeculectomy, or goniosynechialysis in the short- to medium-term outcomes. Additional studies are needed to examine longer periods of follow-up [107]. In selecting IOL power in high hyperopia, studies have compared different formulae to determine the accuracy of formulae predictions. Bai et al. [108] compared the accuracy of Haigis, Hoffer Q, SRKII, Holladay, and SRK/T formulae in 31 eyes and found that the Haigis was the most accurate in IOL in patients with high hyperopia and showed the smallest mean prediction errors (0.37 ± 0.14). The study also found that Hoffer Q was most accurate when measuring axial lengths using A-scan [108]. Comparatively, Kane and Melles [109] conducted a multicenter retrospective case series comparing IOL formulae in 182 eyes using a high power IOL of 30 or more diopters. The formulae compared in this study included Haigis, Hoffer Q, and SRKT, as examined in the previous study, but also included Barrett Universal II, Emmetropia Verifying Optical 2.0, Hill-RBF 2.0, Holladay 1, Holladay 2, Kane, and Olsen. The researchers concluded that the Kane formula had the lowest prediction error within ±0.50 D at 58.8% [109]. Kane and Melles found that the Haigis formulae had a slightly lower prediction error within ±0.50 D at 55.5% [109].

4. Microinvasive glaucoma surgery

The last decade has brought about many new innovations in surgical treatment options and devices for glaucoma. Microinvasive glaucoma surgery (MIGS) is a term used to summarize the surgical interventions that safely and effectively reduce IOP by causing minimal disruption to the normal ocular anatomy, typically through an ab interno approach [110]. The intention of most MIGS procedures is to achieve a lower IOP in glaucoma patients in a shortened surgical time with less postoperative medications needed [110].

The HORIZON study is the largest, prospective, randomized, controlled MIGS pivotal trial that includes data from 556 patients at 38 centers in nine countries [111]. Current data report the 5-year results of this trial with 80% patient follow up comparing cataract surgery alone with combined cataract surgery and intracanalicular stent. The data revealed that after 5 years, cataract surgery in combination with the implantation of the Hydrus microstent was safe, resulting in a sustained lowering of

IOP and reduction in medication use, and reducing the need for additional postoperative glaucoma filtration surgery compared to cataract surgery alone [111]. Cataract patients taking one drop at the time of cataract surgery demonstrated a medication-free rate of 73% following treatment. Of the entire patient cohort, 66% of the patients remained medication-free at the 5-year mark. These findings are pertinent as the data suggest that a reduction in patient adherence to multiple medication regimens can lead to adverse effects [112]. As shown in this trial, MIGS reduces the need for medication and, therefore, lessens the burden of potential adverse effects due to poor patient adherence and can improve patient quality of life. Another key finding of the HORIZON Study is the reduced need for additional surgery. While most patients enrolled in the study had mild glaucoma, the 5-year results showed that those who underwent cataract surgery with the Hydrus microstent were less likely to require invasive incisional glaucoma surgery by more than 2:1 [111]. Visual field analysis showed that patients who underwent cataract surgery and Hydrus had a 47% rate of decreased visual field progression from −0.49 db/year in the cataract surgery alone group to −0.26 db/year in the Hydrus microstent group (P_d = 0.0138) [113]. It is important to note that the patients in this study were limited to POAG eye with age-related cataracts as the only comorbidity. Patients with secondary open-angle glaucoma were not included.

Additional studies have been conducted to determine the efficacy of stents in MIGS procedures. In the 7-year outcomes of the Manchester iStent study, the findings also demonstrated safe outcomes with a maintained reduction in IOP and a decrease in the number of glaucoma medications [114]. The most common complications postoperatively occurred in 3–4% of patients in which the iStent was malpositioned and there was obstruction by blood or iris [114]. Gilmann et al. [115] used in vivo optical coherence tomography to analyze the anatomical and physiological effects of the iStent. The findings suggested that a large portion (45.7%) of iStent inject microstents may be burrowed with the trabeculum and may be related to the increase in device protrusion in the anterior chamber of the eye [115]. Similar results have also been demonstrated with the Kahook dual blade (New World Medical, Rancho Cucamonga, CA). Using the Kahook dual blade (KDB), removal of the trabecular meshwork may be obtained through a minimally invasive approach. This device has demonstrated a clinically significant reduction in IOP as a stand-alone procedure and in combination with cataract surgery [116]. Arnljots and Economou [116] found KDB to offer advantageous reductions in IOP in comparison to the iStent inject and the 1-year results from a prospective study by Elhilali et al. showed KDB to be at least as effective as goniotomy [117]. Additional studies have demonstrated an affordable MIGS option that can be performed with Sinskey hook goniotomy and a 23-, 25-, or 27-gauge straight cystotome [47]. This method is especially useful in resource-poor areas and may be performed at the time of cataract surgery to reduce IOP and restore aqueous outflow to the collector channels [47, 118]. The advantages of this surgery as demonstrated by Tanito include a simple surgical technique, decreased surgery time, less invasiveness to the ocular surface, and no requirement for expensive devices [118].

The complications prominent in trabeculectomy procedures, such as endophthalmitis, bleb, and revisions of bleb, may be avoided in MIGS procedures. The complications associated with MIGS include mispositioning and acutely elevated IOP, which typically occurs in the first month postoperatively and resolves with conservative treatment without the need for further surgery [119]. These complications are infrequent and often transient. As interest in MIGS continues to grow, surgeons continue to utilize this method for effective early intervention in the treatment of glaucoma.

In a recent Iris registry report on MIGS, patients receiving MIGS with and without phacoemulsification showed substantial IOP reduction postoperatively with low complication rates [120]. Overall, MIGS were more likely to fail and require reoperation when performed standalone with nearly a quarter of eyes requiring additional intervention by 2 years [120]. Black patients, eyes with moderate to severe glaucoma, and eyes with higher baseline IOP were more likely to undergo reoperations after MIGS [121].

5. Combined refractive Lensectomy and microinvasive glaucoma surgery

In a study presented at the American Society of Cataract and Refractive Surgery Meeting 2021, Laroche et al. [11] reported the results of clear lensectomy and Hydrus microstent in 134 Black and Afro-Latino patients with glaucoma. The findings revealed that 82.8% of patients were medication free at 1 year. Using the Hodapp-Parrish-Anderson criteria, patients in this study were subdivided into mild, moderate, or advanced glaucoma and presented at an average age of 67.9 years (younger than the typical age for cataract surgery at 73 years). While all patients in this study had a reduction in IOP (mean IOP at 1 year = 13.8 ± 3.1, p = 0.16), the greatest effect in IOP reduction at 1-year follow-up was in patients with mild glaucoma [11]. The greatest reduction in a number of medications was seen in patients with moderate glaucoma, with 92.3% of patients in this group with reduced medication use at 1 year [11]. These findings further emphasized the successful outcomes of early cataract surgery/clear lensectomy combined with MIGS in patients with glaucoma over 50 years of age. Although spikes in IOP (defined as an IOP of >30 mmHg or an increase in IOP >10 mmHg), corneal edema, and hyphema were noted postoperatively, these adverse events were non-vision threatening, self-limiting, and required no further intervention [11].

In a study presented at the World Glaucoma Association 2021 on clear lensectomy and Sinskey hook goniotomy, Laroche et al. [122] detailed the findings collected from 38 eyes with moderately advanced glaucoma measured according to the Humphrey visual field exam. The results of this study demonstrated the effectiveness of combined clear lensectomy and Sinskey hook goniotomy in reducing intraocular pressure and postoperative medication use at 6-months [122]. The baseline medically treated IOP of study participants decreased from 16.45 ± 4.8 mmHg to 13.24 ± 3.0 mmHg over the 6-months and remained at statistically significantly reduced levels [122]. Of the patients treated, 30/38 (78%) no longer used medication at 6 months [122]. High-risk sociodemographic groups, such as Blacks and Afro-Latinos, may face financial burdens that impact medication adherence [123], and therefore can benefit from early combined surgery that reduces the need for further medication use. In the study, transient hyphema occurred in two subjects, which commonly occurs 1 week following goniotomy, and posed no threat to the patients' vision [122]. The Sinskey hook used in this study is also of interest due to its affordable price. The Kahook Dual Blade has been reported by Chen et al. [124] to be the most cost-effective device in terms of cost per reduction of mmHg in intraocular pressure, in comparison to the iStent inject, Trabectome, and Hydrus microstent. The Sinskey hook is readily available as it is a part of most standard cataract sets, making goniotomy more accessible for resource-poor areas and is less costly than the Kahook Dual Blade. This combined therapy can be considered as a safe, first-line treatment for patients with mild to moderate glaucoma by reducing IOP and reducing the need for medication. The use of a Sinskey hook as a more affordable makes this surgery more accessible and affordable in places, such as sub-Saharan Africa, where glaucoma is very prevalent, but resources are limited [125].

Most MIGS procedures do not require an incision to the sclera and are frequently used in combination with phacoemulsification and intraocular lens implantation [110]. The combination of refractive lensectomy and microinvasive glaucoma surgery serves two pivotal purposes in the treatment of POAG—(1) the aging enlarged lens may be removed as the primary contributing cause of glaucoma and (2) physiologic outflow may be restored via collector channels, Schlemm's canal, and the aqueous veins by way of the microinvasive trabecular bypass [5, 113]. This procedure is both efficacious and safe due to the strong outcomes and minimal adverse effects, as previously mentioned above. Therefore, patients over the age of 50 with glaucoma should be considered for the combined treatments of refractive lensectomy and microinvasive trabecular bypass as the first line of treatment, prior to severe disease progression.

Prolonged preoperative glaucoma medication use has been identified as a potential risk factor for the surgical failure of trabeculectomy for reasons that are hypothesized to be related to prolonged inflammation or potential atrophy of the outflow pathway [25]. This outcome further emphasizes the need for early surgery in patients with glaucoma. Additionally, the significant concerns associated with poor medication adherence in long-term glaucoma medical management are addressed in this combined therapy. The need for continuous glaucoma medication is reduced with early intervention with earl cataract surgery/refractive lensectomy with MIGS through the reduction of IOP. Additional long-term studies are needed to determine the extent of the reduction in medication need and burden on patients.

While medical therapy continues to be the first line of treatment for glaucoma, these therapies are now being challenged as the safety, efficacy, advancements, and long-term outcomes of surgical treatments continue to advance. Studies examining the results of combination cataract extraction/refractive lensectomy and MIGS using a microstent have demonstrated a decrease in medication burden and reduction in IOP [125]. As previously mentioned, an additional benefit to these procedures is the affordable price of using tools, such as the Sinskey hook or 23-gauge cystotome, particularly useful in resource-poor areas [126].

6. Conclusion

Glaucoma can lead to irreversible blindness and its severity can affect individuals based on the cost of treatment and impact on quality of life [127]. Although the current first-line treatment options for glaucoma begin with medical management, novel surgical techniques have shown to be effective with long-term efficacy and minimal adverse effects. Additionally, long-term medical management poses the risk of poor patient adherence and may not be sustainable for all individuals. Patients can benefit from early surgical intervention and a reduction in postoperative medication, particularly those in communities at the highest risk for glaucoma and those who have a greater disease burden. Black, Hispanic, and elderly populations are at a disproportionately higher risk of glaucoma [128, 129]. Early treatment interventions and accessible care are imperative to stop glaucoma progression before its severity becomes irreversible [130].

In conclusion, the current standards for the treatment of glaucoma should continue to evolve as innovative and effective surgical techniques are increasing in use in practice. The combined refractive lensectomy and MIGS procedure is a safe and effective early intervention with long-term outcomes that should continue to be further studied. This medical intervention can achieve a decreased IOP in the patient, as well as a reduced medication burden while preserving the visual field. Surgeons should be highly skilled and experienced with very low complication rates.

Author details

Daniel Laroche[1]* and Kara Rickford[2]

1 New York Eye and Ear Infirmary of Mount Sinai, New York, USA

2 New York Medical College, Valhalla, USA

*Address all correspondence to: dlarochemd@aol.com

References

[1] Zhao Y, Fu JL, Li YL, et al. Epidemiology and clinical characteristics of patients with glaucoma: An analysis of hospital data between 2003 and 2012. Indian Journal of Ophthalmology. 2015;**63**(11):825-831. DOI: 10.4103/0301-4738.171963

[2] Liu B, McNally S, Kilpatrick JI, et al. Aging and ocular tissue stiffness in glaucoma. Survey of Ophthalmology. 2018;**63**(1):56-74. DOI: 10.1016/j.survophthal.2017.06.007

[3] Glaucoma Data and Statistics. 2019. Available from: https://www.nei.nih.gov/learn-about-eye-health/outreach-campaigns-and-resources/eye-health-data-and-statistics/glaucoma-data-and-statistics.

[4] Flores-Sanchez BC, Tatham AJ. Acute angle closure glaucoma. British Journal of Hospital Medicine (London, England). 2019;**80**(12):C174-C1C9. DOI: 10.12968/hmed.2019.80.12.C174

[5] Laroche D, Capellan P. The aging lens and glaucoma in persons over 50: Why early cataract surgery/refractive lensectomy and microinvasive trabecular bypass can prevent blindness and cure elevated eye pressure. Journal of the National Medical Association. 2021;**113**(4):471-473. DOI: 10.1016/j.jnma.2021.03.001

[6] Masis M, Mineault PJ, Phan E, et al. The role of phacoemulsification in glaucoma therapy: A systematic review and meta-analysis. Survey of Ophthalmology. 2018;**63**(5):700-710. DOI: 10.1016/j.survophthal.2017.08.006

[7] Leite MT, Sakata LM, Medeiros FA. Managing glaucoma in developing countries. Arquivos Brasileiros de Oftalmologia. 2011;**74**(2):83-84. DOI: 10.1590/s0004-27492011000200001

[8] Hennis A, Wu SY, Nemesure B, et al. Awareness of incident open-angle glaucoma in a population study: The Barbados eye studies. Ophthalmology. 2007;**114**(10):1816-1821. DOI: 10.1016/j.ophtha.2007.06.013

[9] Restrepo NA, Cooke Bailey JN. Primary open-angle glaucoma genetics in African Americans. Current Genetic Medicine Reports. 2017;**5**(4):167-174. DOI: 10.1007/s40142-017-0131-8

[10] Khaw PT, Chiang M, Shah P, et al. Enhanced trabeculectomy: The Moorfields safer surgery system. Developments in Ophthalmology. 2017;**59**:15-35. DOI: 10.1159/000458483

[11] Laroche D, Nkrumah G, Ng C. Clear lensectomy and the hyrdrus stent lower IOP and medication use in black and afro-Latino patients with glaucoma. ASCRS Annual Meeting. Las Vegas, NV: American Society of Cataract and Refractive Surgery. 2021

[12] Ivantis I. Hydrus microstent lowers visual field loss by 47% according to new 5-year pivotal trial data. Clsion PR Newswire. 2021. Available from: https://www.prnewswire.com/news-releases/hydrus-microstent-lowers-visual-field-loss-by-47-according-to-new-5-year-pivotal-trial-data-301423785.html

[13] Types of Glaucoma: National Eye Institute; 2021. Available from: https://www.nei.nih.gov/learn-about-eye-health/eye-conditions-and-diseases/glaucoma/types-glaucoma

[14] Tielsch JM, Katz J, Singh K, et al. A population-based evaluation of glaucoma

screening: The Baltimore eye survey. American Journal of Epidemiology. 1991;**134**(10):1102-1110. DOI: 10.1093/oxfordjournals.aje.a116013

[15] Boland MV, Ervin AM, Friedman DS, et al. Comparative effectiveness of treatments for open-angle glaucoma: A systematic review for the U.S. Preventive Services Task Force. Annals of Internal Medicine. 2013;**158**(4):271-279. DOI: 10.7326/0003-4819-158-4-201302190-00008

[16] American Academy of Ophthalmology Glaucoma Panel, Primary Open Angle Glaucoma: AAO; 2010. Available from: https://www.aao.org/guidelines-browse?filter=Preferred%20Practice%20Patterns&sub=AllPreferredPracticePatterns

[17] Institute NE. Glaucoma Medicines. 2021 July 19. 2021. Available from: https://www.nei.nih.gov/learn-about-eye-health/eye-conditions-and-diseases/glaucoma/glaucoma-medicines

[18] Schuster AK, Erb C, Hoffmann EM, et al. The diagnosis and treatment of glaucoma. Deutsches Ärzteblatt International. 2020;**117**(13):225-234. DOI: 10.3238/arztebl.2020.0225

[19] Netland PA, Landry T, Sullivan EK, et al. Travoprost compared with latanoprost and timolol in patients with open-angle glaucoma or ocular hypertension. American Journal of Ophthalmology. 2001;**132**(4):472-484. DOI: 10.1016/s0002-9394(01)01177-1

[20] Sherwood M, Brandt J, Bimatoprost Study G. Six-month comparison of bimatoprost once-daily and twice-daily with timolol twice-daily in patients with elevated intraocular pressure. Survey of Ophthalmology. 2001;**45**(Suppl. 4): S361-S368. DOI: 10.1016/s0039-6257(01)00219-3

[21] Heijl A, Leske MC, Bengtsson B, et al. Reduction of intraocular pressure and glaucoma progression: Results from the early manifest glaucoma trial. Archives of Ophthalmology. 2002;**120**(10):1268-1279. DOI: 10.1001/archopht.120.10.1268

[22] Shu YH, Wu J, Luong T, et al. Topical medication adherence and visual field progression in open-angle glaucoma: Analysis of a large US health care system. Journal of Glaucoma. 2021;**30**(12):1047-1055. DOI: 10.1097/IJG.0000000000001943

[23] Hollo G, Topouzis F, Fechtner RD. Fixed-combination intraocular pressure-lowering therapy for glaucoma and ocular hypertension: Advantages in clinical practice. Expert Opinion on Pharmacotherapy. 2014;**15**(12):1737-1747. DOI: 10.1517/14656566.2014.936850

[24] Bontzos G, Agiorgiotakis M, E TD. Long-term follow-up of patients receiving intraocular pressure-lowering medications as cataract surgery candidates: A case-control study. Journal of Current Glaucoma Practice. 2017;**11**(3):107-112. DOI: 10.5005/jp-journals-10028-1234

[25] Okuda M, Mori S, Takano F, et al. Association of the prolonged use of anti-glaucoma medications with the surgical failure of ab interno microhook trabeculotomy. Acta Ophthalmologica. 2022;**10**:1111. DOI: 10.1111/aos.15090

[26] Issa de Fendi L, Cena de Oliveira T, Bigheti Pereira C, et al. Additive effect of risk factors for trabeculectomy failure in glaucoma patients: A risk-group from a cohort study. Journal of Glaucoma. 2016;**25**(10):e879-ee83. DOI: 10.1097/IJG.0000000000000490

[27] Broadway DC, Grierson I, O'Brien C, et al. Adverse effects of

topical antiglaucoma medication. II. The outcome of filtration surgery. Archives of Ophthalmology. 1994;**112**(11):1446-1454. DOI: 10.1001/archopht.1994.01090230060021

[28] Landers J, Martin K, Sarkies N, et al. A twenty-year follow-up study of trabeculectomy: Risk factors and outcomes. Ophthalmology. 2012;**119**(4):694-702. DOI: 10.1016/j.ophtha.2011.09.043

[29] Garcia-Posadas L, Contreras-Ruiz L, Soriano-Romani L, et al. Conjunctival goblet cell function: Effect of contact lens Wear and cytokines. Eye & Contact Lens. 2016;**42**(2):83-90. DOI: 10.1097/ICL.0000000000000158

[30] Alvarado JA, Alvarado RG, Yeh RF, et al. A new insight into the cellular regulation of aqueous outflow: How trabecular meshwork endothelial cells drive a mechanism that regulates the permeability of Schlemm's canal endothelial cells. The British Journal of Ophthalmology. 2005;**89**(11):1500-1505. DOI: 10.1136/bjo.2005.081307

[31] Baudoin JP, Viou L, Launay PS, et al. Tangentially migrating neurons assemble a primary cilium that promotes their reorientation to the cortical plate. Neuron. 2012;**76**(6):1108-1122. DOI: 10.1016/j.neuron.2012.10.027

[32] Chae B, Cakiner-Egilmez T, Desai M. Glaucoma medications. Insight. 2013;**38**(1):5-9. quiz 10

[33] Johnson DH, Matsumoto Y. Schlemm's canal becomes smaller after successful filtration surgery. Archives of Ophthalmology. 2000;**118**(9):1251-1256. DOI: 10.1001/archopht.118.9.1251

[34] Samples JR, Singh K, Lin SC, et al. Laser trabeculoplasty for open-angle glaucoma: A report by the american academy of ophthalmology. Ophthalmology. 2011;**118**(11):2296-2302. DOI: 10.1016/j.ophtha.2011.04.037

[35] Conlon R, Saheb H, Ahmed II. Glaucoma treatment trends: A review. Canadian Journal of Ophthalmology. 2017;**52**(1):114-124. DOI: 10.1016/j.jcjo.2016.07.013

[36] Latina MA, Sibayan SA, Shin DH, et al. Q-switched 532-nm Nd:YAG laser trabeculoplasty (selective laser trabeculoplasty): A multicenter, pilot, clinical study. Ophthalmology. 1998;**105**(11):2082-2088; discussion 9-90. DOI: 10.1016/S0161-6420(98)91129-0

[37] Dirani M, Crowston JG, Taylor PS, et al. Economic impact of primary open-angle glaucoma in Australia. Clinical & Experimental Ophthalmology. 2011;**39**(7):623-632. DOI: 10.1111/j.1442-9071.2011.02530.x

[38] Lee R, Hutnik CM. Projected cost comparison of selective laser trabeculoplasty versus glaucoma medication in the Ontario Health Insurance Plan. Canadian Journal of Ophthalmology. 2006;**41**(4):449-456. DOI: 10.1016/S0008-4182(06)80006-2

[39] Wong MO, Lee JW, Choy BN, et al. Systematic review and meta-analysis on the efficacy of selective laser trabeculoplasty in open-angle glaucoma. Survey of Ophthalmology. 2015;**60**(1):36-50. DOI: 10.1016/j.survophthal.2014.06.006

[40] Song J, Lee PP, Epstein DL, et al. High failure rate associated with 180 degrees selective laser trabeculoplasty. Journal of Glaucoma. 2005;**14**(5):400-408. DOI: 10.1097/01.ijg.0000176939.43681.c2

[41] Kuley B, Zheng CX, Zhang QE, et al. Predictors of success in selective

laser trabeculoplasty. Ophthalmology Glaucoma. 2020;**3**(2):97-102. DOI: 10.1016/j.ogla.2019.11.010

[42] Damji KF, Shah KC, Rock WJ, et al. Selective laser trabeculoplasty v argon laser trabeculoplasty: A prospective randomised clinical trial. The British Journal of Ophthalmology. 1999;**83**(6):718-722. DOI: 10.1136/bjo.83.6.718

[43] Gracner T. Intraocular pressure response to selective laser trabeculoplasty in the treatment of primary open-angle glaucoma. Ophthalmologica. 2001;**215**(4):267-270. DOI: 10.1159/000050872

[44] Ticho U, Nesher R. Laser trabeculoplasty in glaucoma. Ten-year evaluation. Archives of Ophthalmology. 1989;**107**(6):844-846. DOI: 10.1001/archopht.1989.01070010866031

[45] Traverso CE, Rolando M, Calabria G, et al. Eye parameters influencing the results of argon laser trabeculoplasty in primary open-angle glaucoma. Ophthalmologica. 1987;**194**(4):174-180. DOI: 10.1159/000309760

[46] Shingleton BJ, Richter CU, Dharma SK, et al. Long-term efficacy of argon laser trabeculoplasty. A 10-year follow-up study. Ophthalmology. 1993;**100**(9):1324-1329. DOI: 10.1016/s0161-6420(93)31480-6

[47] Laroche D, Rickford K, Sakkari S. Case report: Cataract extraction/lensectomy, excisional goniotomy and transscleral cyclophotocoagulation: Affordable combination MIGS for plateau iris glaucoma. Journal of the National Medical Association. 2022;**114**(1):38-41. DOI: 10.1016/j.jnma.2021.12.005

[48] Ramulu PY, Corcoran KJ, Corcoran SL, et al. Utilization of various glaucoma surgeries and procedures in Medicare beneficiaries from 1995 to 2004. Ophthalmology. 2007;**114**(12):2265-2270. DOI: 10.1016/j.ophtha.2007.02.005

[49] Tekeli O, Kose HC. Outcomes of micropulse transscleral cyclophotocoagulation in primary open-angle glaucoma, pseudoexfoliation glaucoma, and secondary glaucoma. European Journal of Ophthalmology. 2021;**31**(3):1113-1121. DOI: 10.1177/1120672120914231

[50] Chamard C, Bachouchi A, Daien V, et al. Efficacy, safety, and retreatment benefit of micropulse transscleral cyclophotocoagulation in glaucoma. Journal of Glaucoma. 2021;**30**(9):781-788. DOI: 10.1097/IJG.0000000000001900

[51] Sanchez FG, Lerner F, Sampaolesi J, et al. Efficacy and safety of micropulse(R) transscleral cyclophotocoagulation in glaucoma. Archivos de la Sociedad Española de Oftalmología. 2018;**93**(12):573-579. DOI: 10.1016/j.oftal.2018.08.003

[52] Lim EJY, Aquino CM, Lun KWX, et al. Efficacy and safety of repeated micropulse transscleral diode cyclophotocoagulation in advanced glaucoma. Journal of Glaucoma. 2021;**30**(7):566-574. DOI: 10.1097/IJG.0000000000001862

[53] Tan AM, Chockalingam M, Aquino MC, et al. Micropulse transscleral diode laser cyclophotocoagulation in the treatment of refractory glaucoma. Clinical & Experimental Ophthalmology. 2010;**38**(3):266-272. DOI: 10.1111/j.1442-9071.2010.02238.x

[54] Pantcheva MB, Kahook MY, Schuman JS, et al. Comparison of acute structural and histopathological changes

of the porcine ciliary processes after endoscopic cyclophotocoagulation and transscleral cyclophotocoagulation. Clinical & Experimental Ophthalmology. 2007;**35**(3):270-274. DOI: 10.1111/j.1442-9071.2006.01415.x

[55] Aquino MC, Barton K, Tan AM, et al. Micropulse versus continuous wave transscleral diode cyclophotocoagulation in refractory glaucoma: A randomized exploratory study. Clinical & Experimental Ophthalmology. 2015;**43**(1):40-46. DOI: 10.1111/ceo.12360

[56] Musch DC, Lichter PR, Guire KE, et al. The collaborative initial glaucoma treatment study: Study design, methods, and baseline characteristics of enrolled patients. Ophthalmology. 1999;**106**(4):653-662. DOI: 10.1016/s0161-6420(99)90147-1

[57] Investigators A. The advanced glaucoma intervention study (AGIS): 11. Risk factors for failure of trabeculectomy and argon laser trabeculoplasty. American Journal of Ophthalmology. 2002;**134**(4):481-498. DOI: 10.1016/s0002-9394(02)01658-6

[58] Comparison of glaucomatous progression between untreated patients with normal-tension glaucoma and patients with therapeutically reduced intraocular pressures. Collaborative Normal-Tension Glaucoma Study Group. American Journal of Ophthalmology. 1998;**126**(4):487-497. DOI: 10.1016/s0002-9394(98)00223-2

[59] Feiner L, Piltz-Seymour JR, Collaborative Initial Glaucoma Treatment S. Collaborative initial glaucoma treatment study: A summary of results to date. Current Opinion in Ophthalmology. 2003;**14**(2):106-111. DOI: 10.1097/00055735-200304000-00010

[60] Chou J, Turalba A, Hoguet A. Surgical innovations in glaucoma: The transition from trabeculectomy to MIGS. International Ophthalmology Clinics. 2017;**57**(4):39-55. DOI: 10.1097/IIO.0000000000000192

[61] Cappelli F, Cutolo CA, Olivari S, et al. Trabeculectomy versus Xen gel implant for the treatment of open-angle glaucoma: A 3-year retrospective analysis. BMJ Open Ophthalmology. 2022;**7**(1):e000830. DOI: 10.1136/bmjophth-2021-000830

[62] Gedde SJ, Schiffman JC, Feuer WJ, et al. Treatment outcomes in the tube versus trabeculectomy (TVT) study after five years of follow-up. American Journal of Ophthalmology. 2012;**153**(5):789-803 e2. DOI: 10.1016/j.ajo.2011.10.026

[63] Chen CW, Huang HT, Bair JS, et al. Trabeculectomy with simultaneous topical application of mitomycin-C in refractory glaucoma. Journal of Ocular Pharmacology. 1990;**6**(3):175-182. DOI: 10.1089/jop.1990.6.175

[64] Heuer DK, Parrish RK 2nd, Gressel MG, et al. 5-Fluorouracil and glaucoma filtering surgery. III. Intermediate follow-up of a pilot study. Ophthalmology. 1986;**93**(12):1537-1546. DOI: 10.1016/s0161-6420(86)33542-5

[65] You YA, Gu YS, Fang CT, et al. Long-term effects of simultaneous subconjunctival and subscleral mitomycin C application in repeat trabeculectomy. Journal of Glaucoma. 2002;**11**(2):110-118. DOI: 10.1097/00061198-200204000-00006

[66] Roy S, Ravinet E, Mermoud A. Baerveldt implant in refractory glaucoma: Long-term results and factors influencing outcome. International Ophthalmology. 2001;**24**(2):93-100. DOI: 10.1023/a:1016335313035

[67] Minckler DS, Francis BA, Hodapp EA, et al. Aqueous shunts in glaucoma: A report by the American Academy of ophthalmology. Ophthalmology. 2008;**115**(6):1089-1098. DOI: 10.1016/j.ophtha.2008.03.031

[68] Christakis PG, Tsai JC, Kalenak JW, et al. The Ahmed versus Baerveldt study: Three-year treatment outcomes. Ophthalmology. 2013;**120**(11):2232-2240. DOI: 10.1016/j.ophtha.2013.04.018

[69] Weiner A, Cohn AD, Balasubramaniam M, et al. Glaucoma tube shunt implantation through the ciliary sulcus in pseudophakic eyes with high risk of corneal decompensation. Journal of Glaucoma. 2010;**19**(6):405-411. DOI: 10.1097/IJG.0b013e3181bdb52d

[70] Laroche D, Sakkari S, Ogunsola T. Combination cataract extraction, goniotomy, Ahmed valve and Retrobulbar tube in a patient with bilateral uveitic glaucoma and Cogan's syndrome. Journal of the National Medical Association. 2022;**113**(6):661-665. DOI: 10.1016/j.jnma.2021.06.003

[71] Tarongoy P, Ho CL, Walton DS. Angle-closure glaucoma: The role of the lens in the pathogenesis, prevention, and treatment. Survey of Ophthalmology. 2009;**54**(2):211-225. DOI: 10.1016/j.survophthal.2008.12.002

[72] Hayashi K, Hayashi H, Nakao F, et al. Changes in anterior chamber angle width and depth after intraocular lens implantation in eyes with glaucoma. Ophthalmology. 2000;**107**(4):698-703. DOI: 10.1016/s0161-6420(00)00007-5

[73] Nonaka A, Kondo T, Kikuchi M, et al. Angle widening and alteration of ciliary process configuration after cataract surgery for primary angle closure. Ophthalmology. 2006;**113**(3):437-441. DOI: 10.1016/j.ophtha.2005.11.018

[74] Azuara-Blanco A, Burr J, Ramsay C, et al. Effectiveness of early lens extraction for the treatment of primary angle-closure glaucoma (EAGLE): A randomised controlled trial. Lancet. 2016;**388**(10052):1389-1397. DOI: 10.1016/S0140-6736(16)30956-4

[75] Tubert D. Nearsightedness: What Is Myopia? American Academy of Ophthalmology2-21. Available from: https://www.aao.org/eye-health/diseases/myopia-nearsightedness

[76] Alio JL, Grzybowski A, Romaniuk D. Refractive lens exchange in modern practice: When and when not to do it? Eye and Vision. 2014;**1**:10. DOI: 10.1186/s40662-014-0010-2

[77] Horgan N, Condon PI, Beatty S. Refractive lens exchange in high myopia: Long term follow up. The British Journal of Ophthalmology. 2005;**89**(6):670-672. DOI: 10.1136/bjo.2004.052720

[78] Arne JL. Phakic intraocular lens implantation versus clear lens extraction in highly myopic eyes of 30- to 50-year-old patients. Journal of Cataract and Refractive Surgery. 2004;**30**(10):2092-2096. DOI: 10.1016/j.jcrs.2004.02.082

[79] Emarah AM, El-Helw MA, Yassin HM. Comparison of clear lens extraction and collamer lens implantation in high myopia. Clinical Ophthalmology. 2010;**4**:447-454. DOI: 10.2147/opth.s11005

[80] Ravalico G, Michieli C, Vattovani O, et al. Retinal detachment after cataract extraction and refractive lens exchange in highly myopic patients. Journal of Cataract and Refractive Surgery. 2003;**29**(1):39-44. DOI: 10.1016/s0886-3350(02)01508-0

[81] Fernandez-Vega L, Alfonso JF, Villacampa T. Clear lens extraction

for the correction of high myopia. Ophthalmology. 2003;**110**(12):2349-2354. DOI: 10.1016/S0161-6420(03)00794-2

[82] Guell JL, Rodriguez-Arenas AF, Gris O, et al. Phacoemulsification of the crystalline lens and implantation of an intraocular lens for the correction of moderate and high myopia: Four-year follow-up. Journal of Cataract and Refractive Surgery. 2003;**29**(1):34-38. DOI: 10.1016/s0886-3350(02)01944-2

[83] Desai P, Minassian DC, Reidy A. National cataract surgery survey 1997-8: A report of the results of the clinical outcomes. The British Journal of Ophthalmology. 1999;**83**(12):1336-1340. DOI: 10.1136/bjo.83.12.1336

[84] DT AJLA. Management of Complications in Refractive Surgery. 2nd ed. Berlin Heildelberg: Springer-Verlag; 2008. pp. 266-269

[85] How will my eye doctor check for retinal detachment?: National Eye Institute; 2020. Available from: https://www.nei.nih.gov/learn-about-eye-health/eye-conditions-and-diseases/retinal-detachmentxw2022

[86] Kaweri L, Wavikar C, James E, et al. Review of current status of refractive lens exchange and role of dysfunctional lens index as its new indication. Indian Journal of Ophthalmology. 2020;**68**(12):2797-2803. DOI: 10.4103/ijo.IJO_2259_20

[87] Fine IH, Hoffman RS, Packer M. Optimizing refractive lens exchange with bimanual microincision phacoemulsification. Journal of Cataract and Refractive Surgery. 2004;**30**(3):550-554. DOI: 10.1016/j.jcrs.2003.07.011

[88] Colin J, Robinet A, Cochener B. Retinal detachment after clear lens extraction for high myopia: Seven-year follow-up. Ophthalmology. 1999;**106**(12):2281-2284; discussion 5. DOI: 10.1016/S0161-6420(99)90526-2

[89] Wilbrandt HR, Wilbrandt TH. Pathogenesis and management of the lens-iris diaphragm retropulsion syndrome during phacoemulsification. Journal of Cataract and Refractive Surgery. 1994;**20**(1):48-53. DOI: 10.1016/s0886-3350(13)80043-0

[90] Gris O, Guell JL, Manero F, et al. Clear lens extraction to correct high myopia. Journal of Cataract and Refractive Surgery. 1996;**22**(6):686-689. DOI: 10.1016/s0886-3350(96)80303-8

[91] Gurnani B, Kaur K. Phacoemulsification. Treasure Island (FL): StatPearls; 2022

[92] Srinivasan B, Leung HY, Cao H, et al. Modern phacoemulsification and intraocular lens implantation (refractive lens exchange) is safe and effective in treating high myopia. Asia-Pacific Journal of Ophthalmology. 2016;**5**(6):438-444. DOI: 10.1097/APO.0000000000000241

[93] Fritch CD. Risk of retinal detachment in myopic eyes after intraocular lens implantation: A 7 year study. Journal of Cataract and Refractive Surgery. 1998;**24**(10):1357-1360. DOI: 10.1016/s0886-3350(98)80228-9

[94] Javitt JC, Vitale S, Canner JK, et al. National outcomes of cataract extraction. I. Retinal detachment after inpatient surgery. Ophthalmology. 1991;**98**(6):895-902. DOI: 10.1016/s0161-6420(91)32204-8

[95] Yoon CH, Shin IS, Kim MK. Trifocal versus bifocal diffractive intraocular lens implantation after cataract surgery or refractive lens exchange: A meta-analysis. Journal of Korean Medical

Science. 2018;**33**(44):e275. DOI: 10.3346/jkms.2018.33.e275

[96] Ge J, Arellano A, Salz J. Surgical correction of hyperopia: Clear lens extraction and laser correction. Ophthalmology Clinics of North America. 2001;**14**(2):301-13, viii

[97] Fink AM, Gore C, Rosen ES. Refractive lensectomy for hyperopia. Ophthalmology. 2000;**107**(8):1540-1548. DOI: 10.1016/s0161-6420(00)00217-7

[98] Alfonso JF, Fernandez-Vega L, Baamonde B, et al. Refractive lens exchange with spherical diffractive intraocular lens implantation after hyperopic laser in situ keratomileusis. Journal of Cataract and Refractive Surgery. 2009;**35**(10):1744-1750. DOI: 10.1016/j.jcrs.2009.04.045

[99] Preetha R, Goel P, Patel N, et al. Clear lens extraction with intraocular lens implantation for hyperopia. Journal of Cataract and Refractive Surgery. 2003;**29**(5):895-899. DOI: 10.1016/s0886-3350(02)01979-x

[100] Hofmann T, Zuberbuhler B, Cervino A, et al. Retinal straylight and complaint scores 18 months after implantation of the AcrySof monofocal and ReSTOR diffractive intraocular lenses. Journal of Refractive Surgery. 2009;**25**(6):485-492. DOI: 10.3928/1081597X-20090512-02

[101] Colin J, Robinet A. Clear lensectomy and implantation of a low-power posterior chamber intraocular lens for correction of high myopia: A four-year follow-up. Ophthalmology. 1997;**104**(1):73-77; discussion 7-8. DOI: 10.1016/s0161-6420(97)30360-1

[102] Yosar JC, Zagora SL, Grigg JR. Cataract surgery in short eyes, including Nanophthalmos: Visual outcomes, complications and refractive results. Clinical Ophthalmology. 2021;**15**:4543-4551. DOI: 10.2147/OPTH.S344465

[103] Schmidt D, Grzybowski A. Vincenz Fukala (1847-1911): Versatile surgeon and early historian of ophthalmology. Survey of Ophthalmology. 2011;**56**(6):550-556. DOI: 10.1016/j.survophthal.2011.04.002

[104] Chang DF. Pars plana vitreous tap for phacoemulsification in the crowded eye. Journal of Cataract and Refractive Surgery. 2001;**27**(12):1911-1914. DOI: 10.1016/s0886-3350(01)00920-8

[105] Rajendrababu S, Babu N, Sinha S, et al. A randomized controlled trial comparing outcomes of cataract surgery in nanophthalmos with and without prophylactic sclerostomy. American Journal of Ophthalmology. 2017;**183**:125-133. DOI: 10.1016/j.ajo.2017.09.008

[106] Zhang Z, Zhang S, Jiang X, et al. Surgical outcomes of 23-gauge transconjunctival pars plana vitrectomy combined with lensectomy for glaucomatous eyes with extremely shallow anterior chamber and cataract. BMC Ophthalmology. 2016;**16**:2. DOI: 10.1186/s12886-015-0179-8

[107] Ong AY, Ng SM, Vedula SS, et al. Lens extraction for chronic angle-closure glaucoma. Cochrane Database of Systematic Reviews. 2021;**3**(3):CD005555. DOI: 10.1002/14651858.CD005555.pub3

[108] Bai L, Zhang ZP, Yi GL, et al. Selection of accurate IOL formula in patients with cataract and high hyperopia. Zhonghua Yan Ke Za Zhi. 2008;**44**(12):1063-1065

[109] Kane JX, Melles RB. Intraocular lens formula comparison in axial hyperopia with a high-power intraocular lens of 30 or more diopters. Journal of Cataract and Refractive Surgery.

2020;**46**(9):1236-1239. DOI: 10.1097/j.jcrs.0000000000000235

[110] Pillunat LE, Erb C, Junemann AG, et al. Micro-invasive glaucoma surgery (MIGS): A review of surgical procedures using stents. Clinical Ophthalmology. 2017;**11**:1583-1600. DOI: 10.2147/OPTH.S135316

[111] Ahmed IIK, De Francesco T, Rhee D, et al. Long term outcomes from the HORIZON randomized trial for a Schlemm's canal microstent in combination cataract and glaucoma surgery. Ophthalmology. 2022;**S0161-6420**(22):00160-9. DOI: 10.1016/j.ophtha.2022.02.021

[112] Ahmed IIK, Rhee DJ, Jones J, et al. Three-year findings of the HORIZON trial: A Schlemm canal microstent for pressure reduction in primary open-angle glaucoma and cataract. Ophthalmology. 2021;**128**(6):857-865. DOI: 10.1016/j.ophtha.2020.11.004

[113] Laroche D, Nkrumah G, Ng C. Real-world efficacy of the Hydrus microstent in black and afro-Latinx patients with glaucoma: A retrospective study. Therapeutic Advances in Ophthalmology. 2020;**12**:2515841420964311. DOI: 10.1177/2515841420964311

[114] Ziaei H, Au L. Manchester iStent study: Long-term 7-year outcomes. Eye (London, England). 2021;**35**(8):2277-2282. DOI: 10.1038/s41433-020-01255-6

[115] Gillmann K, Bravetti GE, Mermoud A, et al. A prospective analysis of iStent inject microstent positioning: Schlemm canal dilatation and intraocular pressure correlations. Journal of Glaucoma. 2019;**28**(7):613-621. DOI: 10.1097/IJG.0000000000001273

[116] Arnljots TS, Economou MA. Kahook dual blade goniotomy vs iStent inject: Long-term results in patients with open-angle glaucoma. Clinical Ophthalmology. 2021;**15**:541-550. DOI: 10.2147/OPTH.S284687

[117] Elhilali HM, El Sayed YM, Elhusseiny AM, et al. Kahook dual blade ab-interno trabeculectomy compared with conventional goniotomy in the treatment of primary congenital glaucoma: 1-year results. Journal of Glaucoma. 2021;**30**(6):526-531. DOI: 10.1097/IJG.0000000000001780

[118] Tanito M. Microhook ab interno trabeculotomy, a novel minimally invasive glaucoma surgery. Clinical Ophthalmology. 2018;**12**:43-48. DOI: 10.2147/OPTH.S152406

[119] Yook E, Vinod K, Panarelli JF. Complications of micro-invasive glaucoma surgery. Current Opinion in Ophthalmology. 2018;**29**(2):147-154. DOI: 10.1097/ICU.0000000000000457

[120] Miller-Ellis EG, Smith O, Croteau-Chonka C, et al. Glaucoma Characteristics for MIGS Utilization: An IRIS Registry Analysis. The Association for Research in Vision and Ophthalmology 2019. Vancouver, CA; 2019

[121] Yang SA, Mitchell W, Hall N, et al. Trends and usage patterns of minimally invasive glaucoma surgery in the United States: IRIS(R) registry analysis 2013-2018. Ophthalmology Glaucoma. 2021;**4**(6):558-568. DOI: 10.1016/j.ogla.2021.03.012

[122] Laroche D, Nkrumah G, Ng C. Clear Lensectomy and affordable Goniotomy with Sinskey hook, lower IOP and medication use in black and afro-Latino patients with glaucoma. World Glaucoma Association Meeting, Japan. 2021

[123] Hu D, Juarez DT, Yeboah M, et al. Interventions to increase medication adherence in African-American and Latino populations: A literature review. Hawai'i Journal of Medicine & Public Health. 2014;**73**(1):11-18

[124] Chen DZ, Sng CCA. Safety and efficacy of microinvasive glaucoma surgery. Journal of Ophthalmology. 2017;**2017**:3182935. DOI: 10.1155/2017/3182935

[125] Egbert PR. Glaucoma in West Africa: A neglected problem. The British Journal of Ophthalmology. 2002;**86**(2):131-132. DOI: 10.1136/bjo.86.2.131

[126] Chen PP, Lin SC, Junk AK, et al. The effect of phacoemulsification on intraocular pressure in glaucoma patients: A report by the American Academy of ophthalmology. Ophthalmology. 2015;**122**(7):1294-1307. DOI: 10.1016/j.ophtha.2015.03.021

[127] Wang Y, Alnwisi S, Ke M. The impact of mild, moderate, and severe visual field loss in glaucoma on patients' quality of life measured via the glaucoma quality of Life-15 questionnaire: A meta-analysis. Medicine (Baltimore). 2017;**96**(48):e8019. DOI: 10.1097/MD.0000000000008019

[128] Shaikh Y, Yu F, Coleman AL. Burden of undetected and untreated glaucoma in the United States. American Journal of Ophthalmology. 2014;**158**(6):1121-9 e1. DOI: 10.1016/j.ajo.2014.08.023

[129] Greenidge KC, Dweck M. Glaucoma in the black population: A problem of blindness. Journal of the National Medical Association. 1988;**80**(12):1305-1309

[130] Tielsch JM, Sommer A, Katz J, et al. Racial variations in the prevalence of primary open-angle glaucoma. The Baltimore Eye Survey. JAMA. 1991;**266**(3):369-374